EVALUATING PUBLIC AND COMMUNITY HEALTH PROGRAMS

MURIEL J. HARRIS

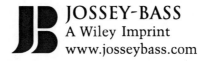

JOSSEY-BASS
A Wiley Imprint
www.josseybass.com

Published by Jossey-Bass
A Wiley Imprint
989 Market Street, San Francisco, CA 94103-1741—www.josseybass.com

Readers should be aware that Internet Web sites offered as citations and/or sources for further information may have changed or disappeared between the time this was written and when it is read.

Limit of Liability/Disclaimer of Warranty: While the publisher and author have used their best efforts in preparing this book, they make no representations or warranties with respect to the accuracy or completeness of the contents of this book and specifically disclaim any implied warranties of merchantability or fitness for a particular purpose. No warranty may be created or extended by sales representatives or written sales materials. The advice and strategies contained herein may not be suitable for your situation. You should consult with a professional where appropriate. Neither the publisher nor author shall be liable for any loss of profit or any other commercial damages, including but not limited to special, incidental, consequential, or other damages.

Jossey-Bass books and products are available through most bookstores. To contact Jossey-Bass directly call our Customer Care Department within the U.S. at 800-956-7739, outside the U.S. at 317-572-3986, or fax 317-572-4002.

Jossey-Bass also publishes its books in a variety of electronic formats. Some content that appears in print may not be available in electronic books.

Library of Congress Cataloging-in-Publication Data

Harris, Muriel J., 1955–
    Evaluating public and community health programs / Muriel J. Harris. — 1st ed.
        p. ; cm.
    Includes bibliographical references and index.
    ISBN 978-0-470-40087-6 (pbk.)
        1.   Public health—Evaluation.   2.   Community health services—Evaluation.   I. Title.
    [DNLM: 1.   Community Health Services—standards.   2.   Program   Evaluation—methods.
    3.   Community-Based Participatory Research.   4.   Data   Collection—methods.
    5.   Evaluation Studies as Topic.   W 84.41 H315e 2010]
    RA440.4.H37 2010
    362.1072—dc22

                                                                                2009044622

10 9 8 7 6 5 4 3 2

CONTENTS

FIGURES AND TABLES

FIGURES

TABLES

PREFACE

In my early career as a public health practitioner I headed a community-based organization that focused on HIV/AIDS prevention for women. I administered lots of surveys to determine the differences in participants' knowledge before and after educational programs. During that period I also assessed a different kind of intervention. In the months leading up to World AIDS Day, we often heard that women felt unable to talk about condoms with their partners and therefore were unable to protect themselves from becoming infected with the virus that causes AIDS. My organization wanted to change that situation and declared World AIDS Day a "No Sex Day," using the print and electronic media to provide information to the public. We encouraged the discussion of HIV/AIDS and abstinence from sex on that day but the use of condoms if couples decided to have sex.

We wanted to know whether our activities leading up to World AIDS Day had any effect on those who heard the programs on radio or television or read articles about our activities in the newspapers. We wanted to know whether women were able to discuss HIV/AIDS with their partners, whether they were able to abstain from having sex, and whether they had used condoms. We wanted to know whether the program effect was different for single women than for married women. We developed a short survey with five simple questions. We did not call what we did an evaluation. It did not have a name. It was just called a questionnaire!

A couple of years later, soon after I completed a situation analysis of homeless children, I was asked to design a drop-in center for this population and to ensure that the project had an evaluation component. Designing the drop-in center was easy. But evaluation was an unfamiliar term to me at the time, and I had lots of questions. What is evaluation? How do you evaluate a drop-in center? How do you know whether you are making a difference for homeless children? Where do you start? I had prepared questionnaires before and after my activities in the past. This evaluation, though, would be different and would test the limits of my experience.

Not long after that and now many years ago, I embarked on a path to learning what that term meant and to developing skills for program evaluation with the support of many wonderful mentors. I now teach program evaluation and take great pleasure in sharing my thoughts and ideas with my students as many of them struggle to learn this challenging subject. As you embark on your journey to learn about evaluating programs, I trust that this book will guide you. You may not know what the term evaluation means, and, like me all those years ago and many of my students now, you are probably still a little wary. No matter where you are in your understanding, my hope is that whether you are a practitioner, a student, or both, you will find this book helpful on your journey and on your path to understanding.

Just as I did many years ago, you probably evaluate what you do all the time without giving it a name. Evaluation is often an unconscious activity that is carried out before choosing among one or many options, both informally and formally. Informal evaluations range from selecting a restaurant for dinner to selecting a course of dishes off the menu. All the decisions you make along the way have implications for the success or failure of the outing. At the end of the evening, you go over the steps you took and decide whether the trip was worth it. If it wasn't, you may decide never to go to that restaurant again. So it is with program evaluation. We assess the resources and activities that went into a program, and then we determine whether the program was worth it to those who participated and to those who funded it.

Evaluation activities occur in a range of work-related settings including community-based organizations, coalitions and partnerships, government-funded entities, the pharmaceutical industry, and the media. Program evaluations assess how an event or activity was conducted, how well it was conducted, and whether it achieved its goal. Evaluation determines the merit of a program or policy, and it forms the basis for decision making.

Evaluation is the cornerstone of program improvement and must be carefully planned and executed to be effective. It helps make the task of assessing the appropriateness of a public health intervention or the success of a program or policy explicit by using appropriate research methods. In evaluation a plan is developed to assess the achievement of program objectives. The plan states the standards against which the intervention will be assessed, the scope of the evaluation, and appropriate tools and approaches for data collection and analysis.

As a further illustration of the evaluation process, let's consider the story of a twenty-four-year-old female who lives in a community not far from where she works. After hearing a lot of talk about the importance of exercising, Antoinette, who works for an evaluation research organization, reached the conclusion that it was a good thing to do, and she decided to check out the neighborhood to see where she could exercise. She knew that she needed to conduct an assessment. She went to the local phone book and found two exercise facilities in her neighborhood.

The following day Antoinette drove by both the gyms and liked what she saw on the outside, but she needed additional information about each facility. She knew that she needed to have a good idea of what she wanted in an exercise facility to be able to make a good judgment. As a result, she sat down and made a list that contained three major categories: the structure and context, content, and expected benefits. Armed with her list of must-haves, which included a well-equipped, safe facility with knowledgeable staff and satisfied customers, she set off to see both facilities. As she approached each facility she looked around at her surroundings and noted the type of building; as she entered she thought about the amount of lighting and the resources that had been put into the facility. She talked to the staff at the desk, the manager, and a trainer. She looked at the equipment and the training programs offered, and finally she talked to a few customers about their experiences and asked whether using the facility had helped them. After a long day Antoinette went home to consider her options. The next morning Antoinette reviewed all the information she had gathered and compared it with her list of must-haves. She compared each facility against her criteria. After analyzing all the data she had collected, she decided that the exercise center that more closely matched her criteria was the best and was the one she would join.

The following week Antoinette set off for the Regent Avenue Gym. She filled out the lengthy membership form, paid her dues, and started her daily exercise routine. Antoinette continually evaluated the program and her surroundings. She monitored the service to determine whether it continued to meet her expectations and all her criteria. After a few weeks in the program Antoinette felt a lot better than she had. She was able to run up stairs, walk longer distances, and overall she just felt better. Her doctor told her that exercising regularly would make her healthier and lower her risk of disease. Antoinette continued to exercise regularly for many years.

Antoinette used a number of approaches to evaluate the Regent Avenue Gym. No one approach or methodology for evaluation fits all situations; so it is important to match the method with the program or policy initiative being evaluated. The stakeholders, who have an interest in the program and the outcome of the evaluation, may influence the type of questions asked, the criteria that are selected, and the evaluation methodologies that are chosen.

There are many opportunities to conduct an evaluation during the life of an intervention, and the approaches to conducting the evaluation in each case will differ. The methods and tools for an evaluation that is conducted during the first few months of a program are different from those used when the program or participation in the program ends and the effectiveness of the program or policy is being assessed. In addition, during the life of the program, evaluation tools and approaches can be used to record program and policy participation and progress.

Evaluation is essentially about making judgments of worth; an evaluation assesses a program's success in achieving the objectives that were established in the beginning. In addition it assesses how well the program was run, who was exposed to the program or policy, and how they benefited from the intervention.

This book presents a model for evaluation and describes the approaches and methods for evaluating community health program and policy interventions. It is aimed at public health and community health students as well as practitioners who are new to program and policy evaluation. This book makes no assumptions of prior knowledge about evaluation. The approach to evaluation that is presented allows for the development of simple or complex evaluation plans while focusing on practical approaches. It encourages a critical thinking and reflective approach with the full involvement of multiple stakeholders throughout the evaluation process. This book provides learners with a systematic, step-by-step approach to program evaluation.

The book is organized into twelve chapters. It discusses the community assessment and the development of the public health initiative as the precursors to the four-step participatory model for evaluation with stakeholders at the center of each component. It frames program evaluation in the context of Community-Based Participatory Research. A case study concludes the book. Additional forms, worksheets, and resources are available for downloading on the publisher's website for the book.

ACKNOWLEDGMENTS

I would like to extend my appreciation to my family, who have supported me in innumerable ways. To D.J. and Benny, I hope this will inspire you to pursue your dreams. Thank you to my mentors, who taught me my first lessons in evaluating programs. Thank you to the organizations that allowed me to develop my evaluation skills through helping others learn evaluation. In the course of doing what we love best, we learn so much. I am grateful that I had the chance to learn from my students, whose patience in learning evaluation through their group projects is a constant inspiration. Thank you to my friends and colleagues, who have continued to encourage me, and to those who reviewed the manuscript and provided important and valuable input and feedback. To my publisher, this dream may never have come true without you. I thank you most sincerely. To each of you who reads this book, I hope you will find much pleasure in learning evaluation.

THE AUTHOR

Muriel J. Harris, PhD, MPH, is an assistant professor at the University of Louisville, School of Public Health and Information Sciences. She also works with the Seattle-based Center for Community Health and Evaluation, part of the Group Health Center for Health Studies, on Kentucky-based evaluation projects.

She developed her interest and her initial practice in public health program evaluation while working in Liberia and Sierra Leone in West Africa. She received her formal training at the Arnold School of Public Health, University of South Carolina. While at the Institute for Families in Society, University of South Carolina, she developed her skills in Empowerment Evaluation and conducted evaluations of a variety of public health programs.

Dr. Harris is a strong supporter of participatory evaluation. In her teaching she supports students as they get real-world experiences from conducting evaluations with community partners. Dr. Harris received the 2008 Delta Omega award for innovative curriculum in public health.

EVALUATING PUBLIC AND COMMUNITY HEALTH PROGRAMS

1

AN INTRODUCTION TO PUBLIC AND COMMUNITY HEALTH EVALUATION

LEARNING OBJECTIVES

- Describe the links among community assessment, program implementation, and program evaluation.

- Describe preassessment evaluations.

- Identify the uses and approaches of evaluation.

- List the principles of Community-Based Participatory Research.

- Explain the ethical and cultural issues in evaluation.

- Describe the value and role of stakeholders in evaluation.

Public health may be assessed by the impact it has on improving the quality of life of people and communities through the elimination or the reduction in the incidence, prevalence, and rates of disease and disability. It should improve conditions and access to resources for healthy living for all people. Public health programs and policies may be instituted at the local, state, national, or international level.

The Committee for the Study of the Future of Public Health defines the mission of public health as "fulfilling society's interest in assuring conditions in which people can be healthy" (Institute of Medicine, 2001, p. 7). Public and community health programs and initiatives exist in order to "do good" and to address social problems or to improve social conditions (Rossi, Lipsey, & Freeman, 2004, p. 17). Public health interventions address social problems or conditions by taking into consideration the underlying factors and core causes of the problem. Within this context, program evaluation determines whether public health program and policy initiatives improve health and quality of life.

Evaluation is often referred to as applied research. Using the word *applied* in the definition lends it certain characteristics that allow it to differ from traditional research in significant ways.

- Evaluation is about a particular initiative. It is generally carried out for the purposes of assessing the initiative, and the results are not generalizable. However, with the scaling up of programs to reach increasingly large segments of the population, and with common outcome expectations and common measures, evaluations can increase their generalizability. Research traditionally aims to produce results that are generalizable to a whole population, place, or setting in a single experiment.

- Evaluations are designed to improve an initiative and to provide information for decision making at the program or policy level; research aims to prove whether there is a cause and effect relationship between two entities in a controlled situation.

- Evaluation questions are generally related to understanding why and how well an intervention worked, as well as to determining whether it worked. Research is much more focused on the end point, on whether an intervention worked.

- Evaluation questions are identified by the stakeholders in collaboration with the evaluators; research questions are usually dictated by the researcher's agenda.

Comparisons of evaluation and research have been associated with a variety of disciplines and approaches (Fitzpatrick, Sanders, & Worthen, 2004). Table 1.1 summarizes the differences.

Some approaches to evaluation, such as those that rely on determining whether goals and objectives are achieved, assess the effects of a program; the judicial approach asks for arguments for and against the program, and program accreditations seek ratings of programs based on a professional judgment of their quality. Consumer-oriented approaches are responsive to stakeholders and encourage their participation. Public health program evaluation utilizes the most appropriate approach for answering the research question, including drawing on social science theories. It incorporates the use

TABLE 1.1.   **A Comparison of Evaluation and Research**

Evaluation	Research
Assesses the particular initiative, and therefore the findings are not generalizable.	Results are generalizable.
Is designed to improve the initiative.	Is designed to prove a relationship.
Focuses on why and how an intervention worked.	Focuses on the end point.
Questions are identified by stakeholders in consultation with the evaluators.	Questions are dictated by the researcher's agenda.
Assesses the value of the initiative even in the face of unexpected results.	Assesses whether the initiative worked.

of the initiative's Theory of Change. A Theory of Change hypothesizes clear and logical links among a program's mission, goal, objectives, and activities.

THE LINKS AMONG COMMUNITY ASSESSMENT, PROGRAM IMPLEMENTATION, AND EVALUATION

When a community or individual identifies a public health problem among a population, steps are taken to understand the problem. These steps constitute community assessments, which define the problem using qualitative and quantitative measures. They assess the extent of the problem, who is most affected, and the individual and environmental factors that may be contributing to and exacerbating the problem. Community assessments determine the activities that will potentially lead to change in the factors that put the population at risk of disease and disability. Programs are planned and implemented based on the findings of the community assessment and the resources available.

The term *initiative* is used in this book to refer to a program or policy intervention that addresses a health or social concern. Details about conducting a community assessment and developing initiatives are discussed in Chapters Two and Three. Examples of initiatives are a program for low-income families to increase their knowledge and skills with regard to accessing health care and an after-school program to improve physical fitness. Programs may also modify the environment to improve access to conditions that support health, such as improving conditions for walking in a community or improving access to fresh produce. Initiatives can also develop or change public policy so that more people can have health insurance and improved access to health care.

An initiative may have multiple activities, programs, or policies. One example is prevention of the onset of diabetes, which requires a multipronged intervention for those at risk. Individual components that constitute the initiative may include physical activity, diet control, case management, outreach education, and policies that increase the availability of fresh produce. Evaluating a multipronged initiative requires assessing both process and outcomes for each component as well as assessing the overall effect of the initiative on preventing diabetes among the target population.

Evaluation activities may occur at multiple points on a continuum, from planning the initiative, through implementation, to assessing the effect on the populations served and meeting the goals outlined in the Healthy People objectives (U.S. Department of Health and Human Services, 2000). The Healthy People documents identify the most significant preventable threats to health and establish national goals to reduce these threats. Individuals, groups, and organizations are encouraged to integrate the Healthy People objectives into the development of initiatives. In addition, businesses can use the framework to build work-site health-promotion activities; schools and colleges can undertake programs and activities to improve the health of students and staff. Health care providers can encourage their patients to pursue healthy lifestyles; community-based organizations and civic and faith-based organizations can develop initiatives to address health issues in a community, especially among hard-to-reach populations, and to ensure that everybody has access to information and resources for healthy living.

Determining the effectiveness of the implementation of programs and policies and the impact of such initiatives on the population that is reached is the task of program- or policy-evaluation activities. Although evaluation activities may use different approaches, their function is similar across disciplines. Formative evaluation is the appropriate approach during the program planning and development phase of an initiative; process monitoring and evaluation are useful during the implementation phase and when the goal of the evaluation is to understand what went into the program and how well it is being implemented.

Outcome evaluations are carried out after programs have been in place for a time and are considered stable; such an evaluation can assess the effect of a program or policy on individuals or a community. Outcome evaluation aims to understand whether a program was effective and achieved what it set out to accomplish. Impact evaluation is the last stage of the evaluation continuum. It is used when multiple programs and policy initiatives affect the quality of life of a large population over a long period. Multiple interventions on the population or subpopulation are assessed for changes in quality of life and for the incidence and prevalence of disease or disability. Discussions of impact evaluation may be found in other texts. Figure 1.1 illustrates the context of evaluation; the specific kinds of evaluation are discussed in detail in the next section.

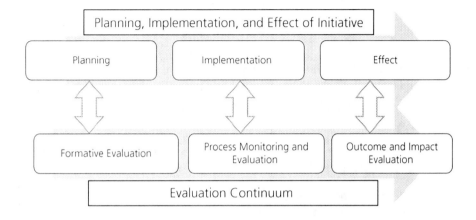

FIGURE 1.1.   *Evaluation in Context*

OVERVIEW OF EVALUATION

Rossi et al. (2004) describe evaluation as "the use of social research methods to systematically investigate the effectiveness of social intervention programs in ways that are adapted to their political and organizational environments and are designed to inform social action to inform social conditions" (p. 16). In addition, these authors caution that evaluation provides the best information possible under conditions that involve a political process of balancing interests and reaching decisions (p. 419).

Evaluation is the cornerstone for improving public health programs and is conducted for the purpose of making a judgment of a program's worth or value. Evaluation incorporates steps that specify and describe the activities and the process of evaluation; the initiative and why it is being evaluated; the measures needed to assess the inputs, outputs, and outcomes; and the methodology for collecting the information (data). In addition, an evaluation analyzes data and disseminates results in ways that ensure that the evaluation is useful to the stakeholders.

PREASSESSMENT EVALUATIONS

One major assumption in evaluating an initiative is that it was well planned and fully implemented. This, however, is not always the case, and the evaluation team may then find it must balance the expense associated with undertaking the evaluation with the likely result of the evaluation. The question becomes, In undertaking this evaluation will we be able to provide useful information to the stakeholder for decision making or program improvement? If the answer is no, the initiative may not be ready for an evaluation. If the answer is yes, consultation may be necessary with regard to various aspects of the evaluation for which stakeholder participation is critical. Preassessment thus may be thought of as a feasibility study of the initiative's readiness to be evaluated. Components of a feasibility evaluation may include:

- Assessing the readiness of executives, staff, and stakeholders to support an evaluation and to use the results

- Determining whether the stated goals and objectives are clear and reflect the intended direction of the organization

- Assessing the logic of the program and its ability to achieve the stated goal and objectives given the initiative's activities and resources

- Assessing whether data collected of the program's implementation activities are likely to be suitable for showing the effects of the program

- Assessing whether processes exist or can be developed to provide sufficient information to assess the program's activities, outputs, and outcomes

- Assessing access to program participants, program staff, and other stakeholders

- Assessing the logistics and resources available to conduct an evaluation

Whether preassessment is completed formally or informally, the outcome may be either that the evaluation is able to go ahead or that it has to be delayed until various conditions are met. Meeting the conditions may require anything from developing a set of data-management and evaluation tools that allow for appropriate and adequate data collection to taking far-reaching measures such as collecting baseline data and restructuring the initiative. Such actions ensure that the program has the components and tools essential for undertaking an appropriate and meaningful evaluation in the future.

One of the detailed tasks in carrying out a preassessment is to work with the organization to understand its contexts and programs, the epidemiological and community data-based rationale, and the resources for the intervention. The evaluator identifies the intervention components, creates a Theory of Change model, and determines the existence (or nonexistence) of specific, measurable, realistic, achievable, and time-oriented short-term, intermediate, and long-term outcome objectives.

COMMUNITY-BASED PARTICIPATORY RESEARCH

A fundamental principle of evaluation is that the evaluation team has a responsibility not only to the profession but to the community. The American Evaluation Association (2008, p. 234) reminds us:

Evaluators articulate and take into account the diversity of general and public interests and values and thus should: 1) include relevant perspectives and interests of the full range of stakeholders, 2) consider not only immediate operations and outcomes of the evaluation but also the broad assumptions, implications and potential side effects,

3) allow stakeholders access to and actively disseminate evaluative information and present evaluation results in understandable forms that respect people and honor promises of confidentiality, 4) maintain the balance between client and stakeholder needs and interests, and 5) take into account the public interest and good, going beyond analysis of particular stakeholder needs and interests to consider the welfare of society as a whole.

A participatory model for evaluation views evaluation as a team effort that involves people internal and external to the organization with varying levels of evaluation expertise in a power-sharing and co-learning relationship.

Patton (2008, p. 175) identifies nine principles of participatory evaluation:

1. The process involves participants in learning skills.

2. Participants own the evaluation and are active in the process.

3. Participants focus the evaluation on what they consider important.

4. Participants work together as a group.

5. The whole evaluation process is understandable and meaningful to the participants.

6. Accountability to oneself and to others is valued and supported.

7. The perspectives and expertise of all persons are recognized and valued.

8. The evaluator facilitates the process and is a collaborator and a resource for the team.

9. The status of the evaluator relative to the team is minimized (to allow equitable participation).

A participatory model for evaluation embraces the stakeholders in the process and utilizes approaches to help the organization develop the capacity to evaluate its own programs and institute program improvement (Fetterman, Kaftarian, & Wandersman, 1996). By adopting Community-Based Participatory Research (Israel, Eng, & Parker, 2005), evaluation emphasizes self-determination, learning, and empowerment, and incorporates both qualitative and quantitative methods for data collection. It under-scores the value of including those who have a vested interest in the programs and their communities in the process (Minkler, 2007).

The Community-Based Participatory Research approach (Israel, Eng, Schulz, & Parker 2005) proposes nine guiding principles for collaboration; these guidelines are easily incorporated into participatory program evaluation of public health initiatives. Community-Based Participatory Research

1. acknowledges community as a unit of identity in which people have membership; it may be identified as a geographical area or a group of individuals

2. builds on strengths and resources of the community and utilizes them to address the needs of the community

3. facilitates a collaborative, equitable partnership in all phases of research, involving an empowering and power-sharing process that attends to social inequalities with open communication among all partners and an equitable share in the decision making

4. fosters co-learning and capacity building among all partners with a recognition that people bring a variety of skills, expertise, and experience to the process

5. integrates and achieves a balance between knowledge generation and intervention for the mutual benefit of all partners with the translation of research findings into action

6. focuses on the local relevance of public health problems from an ecological perspective that addresses the multiple determinants of health including biological, social, economic, cultural, and physical factors

7. involves systems development using a cyclical and iterative process that includes all the stages of the research process from assessing and identifying the problem to action

8. disseminates results to all partners and involves them in the wide dissemination of results in ways that are respectful

9. involves a long-term process and commitment to sustainability in order to build trust and have the ability to address multiple determinants of health over an extended period (Israel et al., 2005, pp. 7–9)

Important outcomes of Community-Based Participatory Research approaches are building community infrastructure and community capacity, knowledge, and skills (O'Fallon & Dearry, 2002).

THE PARTICIPATORY MODEL FOR EVALUATION

The Participatory Model for Evaluation is based on the Framework for Program Evaluation (Milstein, Wetterhall, & Group, 2000), which has six evaluation steps (Figure 1.2).

The Participatory Model for Evaluation, adopted in this book, incorporates Community-Based Participatory Research principles (Israel et al., 2005) and supports a collaborative, equitable partnership in all phases of the evaluation process. It fosters co-learning and capacity building while acknowledging and utilizing existing experience and expertise. It incorporates all the elements of the evaluation process but does so in a flexible and simplified way. It recognizes the often iterative and integrative nature of evaluation in designing the evaluation; collecting, analyzing, and interpreting the data; and reporting the findings. It links the evaluation process to community assessment and program planning and implementation in a deliberative and iterative way. Stakeholders' active participation in the process provides flexibility in the evaluation

FIGURE 1.2.   *Framework for Program Evaluation in Public Health*

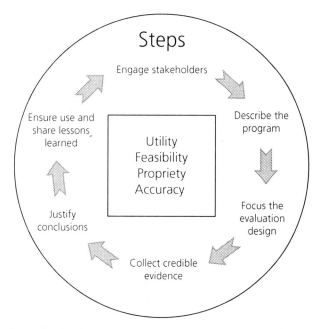

From Milstein, Wetterhall, & Group (2000).

and allows it to be customizable to the users' needs. Because conducting an evaluation depends on a thorough knowledge and understanding of a program's development, this book provides an overview of these critical precursors to evaluation, the community assessment, and developing programs for evaluation. This model recognizes the dynamic nature of programs and the changing needs of the evaluation over time, hence the cyclical nature of the process.

The Participatory Model for Evaluation (Figure 1.3) used to evaluate public health community or policy initiatives recognizes that the community assessment and the public health initiative are precursors to an evaluation. The Participatory Model for Evaluation consists of four major steps:

1. Design the evaluation.

2. Collect the data.

3. Analyze and interpret the data.

4. Report the findings.

In this model of evaluation, stakeholders who have a vested interest in the program's development, implementation, or results are part of the evaluation team and

FIGURE 1.3. *The Participatory Model for Evaluation*

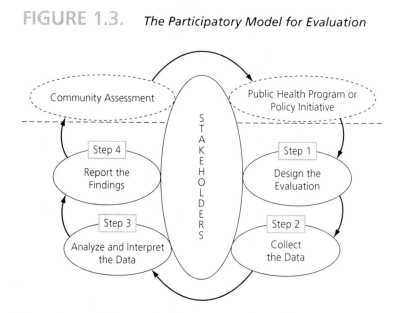

involved in each step of the evaluation process. In addition to acknowledging the inclusion of stakeholders as good practice in evaluation, the Public Health Leadership Society (2002) recognizes their inclusion as being ethical. Its principle 3 states that public health "policies, programs, and priorities should be developed and evaluated through processes that ensure an opportunity for input from community members" (p. 4). Stakeholders provide multiple perspectives and a deep understanding of the cultural context in which an initiative is developed and an evaluation conducted.

The Evaluators

The team is led by an experienced evaluator who may be internal or external to the organization. Historically, the evaluator has been an outsider who comes in to give an independent, "unbiased" review of the initiative. More recently, agencies and large nonprofit organizations have hired in-house evaluators or modified the roles of staff to provide evaluation and thereby strengthen the overall capacity of the organization. A significant advantage is that the agency may be able to have a more sustained evaluation conducted at lower cost. Irrespective of the approach used, participatory models include stakeholders as part of the evaluation design and implementation in order to facilitate the use of the findings.

There are advantages and disadvantages to choosing an internal or an external evaluator. An internal person who has the expertise to conduct an evaluation and who knows the program well may also have easy access to materials, logistics, resources, and data. However, internal evaluators are often too busy, may be less objective than external people, and may have limited expertise.

An external evaluator is often viewed as being more credible, more objective, and better able to offer additional insights and to serve as a facilitator than someone from inside the organization. An external person may also be able to provide additional resources. Alternatively, external evaluators may not know the program, policies, and procedures of the organization, may not understand the program context, and may be perceived as adversarial and an imposition.

Whether an evaluator is internal or external, the person who has the primary responsibility for the evaluation should have these essential competencies:

- Know and maintain professional norms and values, including evaluation standards and principles

- Use expertise in the technical aspects of evaluation such as design, measurement, data analysis, interpretation, and sharing results

- Use situational analysis, understand and attend to contextual and political issues of an evaluation

- Understand the nuts and bolts of evaluation, including contract negotiation, budgeting, and identifying and coordinating needed resources for a timely evaluation

- Be reflective regarding one's practice and be aware of one's expertise as well as the need for professional growth

- Have interpersonal competence in written communication and the cross-cultural skills needed to work with diverse groups of stakeholders (Ghere, King, Stevahn, & Minnema, 2006; King, Stevahn, Ghere, & Minnema, 2001)

In addition, five ethical principles of program evaluation were adopted and ratified by the American Evaluation Association. These principles reflect the fundamental ethical principles of autonomy, nonmaleficence, beneficence, justice, and fidelity (Veach, 1997) and as such provide an ethical compass for action and decision making throughout the evaluation process. These principles are the following:

1. *Systematic inquiry:* Evaluators conduct systematic, data-based inquiries. They adhere to the highest technical standards; explore the shortcomings and strengths of evaluation questions and approaches; communicate the approaches, methods, and limitations of the evaluation accurately; and allow others to be able to understand, interpret, and critique their work.

2. *Competence:* Evaluators provide competent performance to stakeholders. They ensure that the evaluation team possesses the knowledge, skills, and experience required; that it demonstrates cultural competence; practices within its limits; and continuously provides the highest level of performance.

3. *Integrity/honesty:* Evaluators display honesty and integrity in their own behavior and attempt to ensure the honesty of the entire evaluation process. They negotiate honestly, disclose any conflicts of interest and values and any sources of financial support. They disclose changes to the evaluation, resolve any concerns, accurately represent their findings, and attempt to prevent any misuse of those findings.

4. *Respect for people:* Evaluators respect the security, dignity, and worth of respondents, program participants, clients, and other stakeholders. They understand the context of the evaluation, abide by ethical standards, conduct the evaluation and communicate results in a way that respects the stakeholders' dignity and worth, fosters social equity, and takes into account all persons.

5. *Responsibilities for general and public welfare:* Evaluators articulate and take into account the diversity of general and public values that may be related to the evaluation. They include relevant perspectives, consider also the side effects, and allow stakeholders to present the results in appropriate forms that respect confidentiality, take into account the public interest, and consider the welfare of society as a whole (American Evaluation Association, 2008, pp. 233–234).

(The full text of the American Evaluation Association Guiding Principles for Evaluators is available at http://www.eval.org.)

The second principle, competence, refers to providing skilled evaluation. "Evaluators should possess (or ensure that the evaluation team possesses) the education, abilities, skills and experience appropriate to undertake the tasks proposed by the evaluation" (American Evaluation Association, 2008, p. 233). In addition the evaluation team develops cross-cultural skills in order to understand the culture in which both the initiative and the evaluation are embedded (Ghere et al., 2006; King et al., 2001).

The Stakeholders

Stakeholders who are identified to be part of the evaluation team are individuals, groups, or organizations that have a significant interest in how well a program functions (Rossi et al., 2004). Involving stakeholders allows the initiative to be viewed in the appropriate administrative, epidemiological, political, and sociocultural perspectives.

Stakeholders provide the funding for the program, management, or oversight or are participants in the program and benefit from program activities. In addition, some have an interest in the program but do not have any specific role in the organization and its initiatives. It is equally important to engage those community members who are not supportive of the initiative to understand their concerns and the competition that the organization faces. Involving multiple stakeholders in the process enhances the credibility of the evaluation, ensures that the appropriate voices are heard, and gives stakeholders ownership in the evaluation.

A stakeholder analysis will help identify the stakeholders who are associated with the program, their interest in the program, and their likely contribution to the evaluation tasks. The stakeholder analysis is conducted at the start and throughout the evaluation process to ensure that the right people are included at critical points, from developing the evaluation design to reporting the results. During the evaluation the roles of the stakeholders change as they go in and out of the process and participate as is appropriate for their interest and expertise. Stakeholders in a public health evaluation could include:

- The board of directors of the organization that has requested the evaluation to determine whether the organization is meeting the requirements for continued funding

- The board of directors of a foundation that provides community grants and wants to be sure its grants are making a difference in achieving strategic goals

- The executive director, who provides overall oversight and management for the program

- The project manager, who provides the day-to-day management of staff implementing the program or the policy

- Staff providing services to clients

- Staff supervising logistical services

- Persons receiving services who meet the criteria for the intended population sample

- Persons who are affected in any way by the services or policies

- Persons in the larger community who have an interest in the program's success

Ideally stakeholders are involved in the evaluation from the start and throughout the process. In addition to their invaluable input into understanding program development and implementation, stakeholders have critical roles and responsibilities that include providing

- access to files, reports, and publications

- administrative and logistical support

- access to other stakeholders as necessary for data collection

- support in implementing the evaluation plan

- insights into the results and interpretation of the data analysis

- support in disseminating the interim and final reports

Keeping stakeholders engaged in the evaluation process involves developing meaningful relationships with them. Relationship development may be facilitated by understanding some of their issues, understanding the cultural and power issues that exist, and working to develop a trusting and ethical relationship.

CULTURAL CONSIDERATIONS IN EVALUATION

With the changing demographics of most countries, states, counties, cities, and neighborhoods, being sensitive to other cultures is important and may make the difference between an evaluation that produces useful findings and one that does not. It may be the difference between having a set of behaviors, attitudes, and practices that enables effective work and not being effective. Knowing there are differences among cultures and yet avoiding value judgments that undermine the integrity of a people is an underlying principle of cross-cultural engagement. Appreciating and embracing cultures different from our own facilitates an environment conducive to each person's growth and development.

Although there are many definitions of culture, it is generally thought to refer to a set of beliefs, traditions, and behavior that apply to a particular group of people. Cultural groups may be identified based on age, gender, religion, country of origin, race or ethnicity, sexual orientation, disability, family background, language, food preference, employment, or neighborhood community. These characteristics influence societal traditions, thought patterns, processes, and traditions. Sector (1995, p. 68) defines culture as "the sum of beliefs, practices, habits, likes, dislikes, norms, customs, rituals, and so forth that we learned from our families during the years of socialization."

Societal customs and traditions are passed through multiple generations and may include the way members of the group dress, sing, and dance or how they perceive and respond to the world around them. Traditions are passed down by word of mouth during periods of storytelling or less deliberately when societies perform traditions year after year. Native Americans, for example, have many traditions that define their culture as do Africans and Asians both in their native areas and in the Diaspora.

Certain practices are unique to a cultural group, but often we find similar traditions across groups. It is fascinating to observe that black populations that live in America, the Caribbean, and Canada have traditions and thought patterns similar to those of blacks who still live in Africa even though they have been separated for many generations. As cultures have become integrated through immigration and intermarriage, we see changes in cultural practices. Societies continue to eliminate those practices that are harmful and retain those that speak to the core values of their people.

Because culture gives people unique perspectives and often unique ways of doing, developing the knowledge and skills to work cross-culturally is critical to effective practice. To be able to fully appreciate and consider another person's culture, it is important to learn about that culture. Learning requires humility of spirit, openness and honesty, patience and a willingness to share what we know with others.

When we take the culture of the people around us into consideration, we demonstrate

▨   a respect for others

▨   a willingness to listen to the perspective of others and to respect their views

▨   a willingness to learn

Culture plays an important role in program evaluation. Cultural context guides the methods and approaches that are used throughout the process as well as the interpretation of the results and how the conclusions are drawn. As a result, culture influences the validity of the evaluation findings (Johnson, Kirkhart, Madison, Noley, & Solano-Flores, 2008). Aspects of the evaluation process that culture affects include:

- How the evaluation questions are asked

- The selection of the data sources

- The methods and approaches used to collect the evaluation data

- The techniques used in the evaluation

- The methods and approaches used in communication of the results (Kirkhart, 2005)

Standards of cultural competence have often been used to define the expectations of those working with a diverse population. Cultural competence incorporates the hope that the workforce has the knowledge, attitudes, and skills necessary to understand the beliefs, behaviors, and practices of the population being served. It is also necessary that they have demographic characteristics similar to those of the receivers of the services or, in some cases, that they simply be able to provide language-translation services.

Cultural competence has been defined in multiple ways. Batancourt, Green, Carillo, and Ananeh-Firenpong (2003, p. 294) suggest that "[cultural competence] acknowledges and incorporates at all levels, the importance of culture, assessment of cross-cultural relations, vigilance towards the dynamics that result from cultural differences, expansion of cultural knowledge, and adaptation of services to meet culturally unique needs." Perez and Luquis (2008) identify three characteristics that are conducive to reaching mutual goals: cultural desire (the desire to work in a multicultural society), cultural awareness, and cultural sensitivity. Cultural competence may be characterized as knowledge, attitudes, and values that, when applied systematically, lead to the empowerment of others irrespective of their culture.

In recognizing the significance of paying attention to culture and valuing the input and expertise of others, the American Evaluation Association's Guiding Principles for Evaluators (2008, item D.6) reads, "Understand, respect, and take into account differences among stakeholders such as culture, religion, disability, age and sexual orientation and ethnicity." To do so, one must be culturally competent. Cultural competence in evaluation means

- being open, respectful, and appreciative of another's culture

- acknowledging the value of other cultures

- recognizing culturally based understandings

- incorporating cultural understanding into each step of the evaluation process

Cultural competence is a journey and does not have a discrete end point because we never really become competent in another person's culture; however, cultural humility and the ability to listen to people from other cultures and to evaluate ourselves are important characteristics of evaluators who are culturally competent (Tervalon & Murray-Garcia, 1998). Cultural humility includes understanding the impact of one's professional culture, which helps shape the relationship between the evaluator and the stakeholders. An important result of a relationship where there is cultural humility is likely to be full and equitable participation for all stakeholders.

The American Evaluation Association standards include two guiding competencies for evaluators that focus on cultural understanding (2008, items B.2 and D.14):

1. Demonstrate a sufficient level of cultural competence to ensure recognition, accurate interpretation, and respect for diversity

2. Become acquainted with and respect differences among participants, including their culture, religion, gender, disability, age, sexual orientation, and ethnicity

One of the earliest phases in the development of cultural competence is acquiring cultural sensitivity. In evaluation, cultural sensitivity dictates that the evaluation team

▓ shed light on why a particular program works from the perspective of the participants and the stakeholders

▓ design an appropriate evaluation process

▓ interpret data with sensitivity and understanding

▓ promote social justice and equity

In the application of cultural understanding to evaluation, Kirkhart (2005) describes multicultural validity in evaluation research as the recognition and application of understanding of cultural context to increase the validity of the research process from the formation of the evaluation question to the communication of findings. Kirkhart (2005) identifies five ways that culture influences the validity of an evaluation:

1. *Interpersonal* approaches assess the quality of the interactions between and among participants in the evaluation process.

2. *Consequential* approaches assess the social consequences of understandings and judgments and the actions taken based on them.

3. *Methodological* approaches assess the cultural appropriateness of measurement tools and the cultural congruence of evaluation designs.

4. *Theoretical* approaches assess the cultural congruence of theoretical perspectives underlying the program, the evaluation, and the assumptions of validity.

5. *Experiential* approaches assess congruence with the lived experience of participants in the program and in the evaluation process.

In integrating cultural perspectives into its work, the United Nations Population Fund identified twenty-four tips for culturally sensitive programming (United Nations Population Fund, n.d.). Drawing on that work, I list here ten of the tips that mirror the principles guiding the implementation of the Participatory Model for Evaluation:

1. Invest time in knowing the culture in which you are operating.

2. Hear what the community has to say.

3. Demonstrate respect.

4. Be inclusive.

5. Honor commitments.

6. Find common ground.

7. Build community capacity.

8. Let people do what they do best.

9. Provide solid evidence.

10. Rely on the objectivity of science.

(A full list of the tips may be found at http://www.unfpa.org/culture/24/cover.htm.)

The Participatory Model for Evaluation incorporates an empowerment philosophy that integrates a cultural perspective and leaves the community with knowledge, skills, and an increased capacity and ability to conduct its own evaluation by including a community-based participatory research philosophy.

SUMMARY

- Evaluation is conducted by a team that consists of evaluators and stakeholders who share responsibility for the evaluation from the start of the process to completing the report and presenting the results.

- The Participatory Model for Evaluation considers the community assessment and the public health program or policy initiative as precursors to evaluation.

- Community-Based Participatory Research fosters the involvement of stakeholders in all aspects of the evaluation from describing the initiative's context to writing the final evaluation report.

- The guiding principles for performing evaluation are systematic inquiry, competence, integrity, respect for persons, and responsibility for the public welfare.

- Culture refers to a set of beliefs, traditions, and behavior of a group of people that may be identified by personal characteristics, geographical area, or common interests.

DISCUSSION QUESTIONS AND ACTIVITIES

1. Define *evaluation*. Explain what evaluation means in your own words. Provide an example of an evaluation and draw a graph, picture, or in other ways illustrate what evaluation means to you.

2. Locate and read at least one article that uses a participatory approach to evaluation and another that does not use that approach. Summarize the main points of each article and discuss differences between the approaches.

3. Identify a culture different from your own. Which of the characteristics you know about in that culture are similar to those of your culture and which are different from those of your own culture? Make a list. Now, do a literature search to learn more about the culture you selected and write a one-to-two page summary of your findings.

4. Go to the full text of the Guiding Principles for Evaluators at www.eval.org. Discuss Guiding Principle D in your own words. Identify and review Institutional Review Board requirements usually found in agencies, universities, and colleges, or in research institutions. How is Guiding Principle D reflected in the requirements for the protection of human subjects? Note: Institutional Review Boards are sometimes referred to as Ethics Committees or Ethical Review Boards.

KEY TERMS

Community-Based Participatory Research

community health

cultural competence

ethical principles in evaluation

evaluation

initiative

participatory evaluation

Participatory Model for Evaluation

preassessment evaluation

public health

stakeholders

CHAPTER

2

THE COMMUNITY ASSESSMENT

AN OVERVIEW

LEARNING OBJECTIVES

▪ Describe the relationship of community assessment to the implementation of public and community health programs and to program evaluation.

▪ Identify and describe approaches to conducting a community assessment.

▪ Describe a literature review as a component of the community assessment.

▪ Explain the value and role of stakeholders in conducting a community assessment.

Public health concerns such as high or detectable rates of morbidity or mortality among a specified population may result in attempts to address the problem by proposing solutions and developing interventions. From the perspective of an evaluator, the intervention that is developed requires appraisal on two levels. First, it requires that the problem be specified: Who are affected? Why are they affected? How many members of the community are affected? Second, it requires an understanding of the assets and resources available for addressing the problem.

A community assessment determines the extent of the problem and proposes the most feasible, viable, and effective solution or combination of solutions to address the problem adequately and appropriately. A community assessment depicts the perceived and actual needs of a given population and their assets and resources for the development of a public health initiative. The community assessment precedes the evaluation process in the Participatory Model for Evaluation, as shown in Figure 2.1. This chapter provides an overview of the community assessment.

Community assessments are an important and integral part of program planning and are conducted with the community as the focus (Sharpe, Greany, Lee, & Royce, 2005). The community may be a geographical, faith, racial/ethnic, school, professional, or cultural community, to name a few. The community assessment is part of a cyclical and iterative process and precedes the selection, development, and implementation of the initiative (Figure 2.2). A community assessment may also be required following an evaluation to identify additional community needs, assets, and priorities and to determine next steps for program development. The assessment may, in addition, herald the refinement of the initiative or the start of a new one.

Why conduct a community assessment?

FIGURE 2.1. *The Community Assessment as a Component of the Participatory Model for Evaluation*

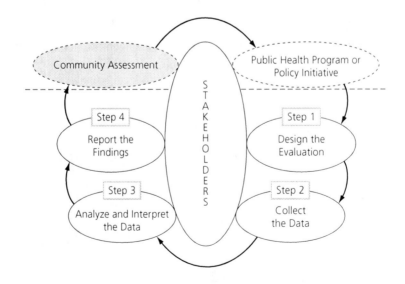

- To identify where the problem is most prevalent

- To identify the people or groups of people who are most affected by the problem or involved with the problem

- To identify the factors that produce the problem at the individual, physical, and/or social-environmental level

- To assess individual and community needs and aspirations

- To assess the community's readiness to address the problem

- To assess the level of resources available within the community to address the problem

- To obtain data that can be used to support the development of the initiative and provide the baseline against which any changes in the problem may be assessed

A community assessment can also be described as a situation analysis that may produce an extensive appraisal of the affected community.

For the assessment process to be empowering and to benefit the community, Hancock and Minkler (2007) advocate that it be "of the community, by the community and for the community" (p. 138). An important aspect of this approach is that the community is involved in the process; the findings are provided to the community and can then be utilized by the community for decision making.

Because a participatory process is likely to result in the development of sustainable, community-driven solutions to the problem, Hancock and Minkler (2007, p. 144) suggest incorporating questions that are important to the community in the assessment process. Such questions include:

- What are the history, economic welfare, and leadership of the community?

- What individual characteristics, behaviors, and practices contribute to the problem?

- Do people have access to basic amenities that support healthy living?

- To what extent do equity and fairness exist in the community?

- What is the nature of civic associations, and to what extent do they support all facets of community life?

FIGURE 2.2. *The Community Assessment, the Initiative, and the Evaluation*

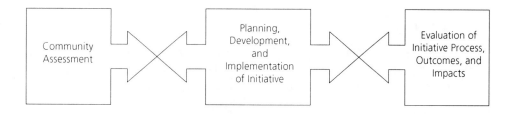

- How do the social and physical environments affect the health and well-being of the community?

- What is currently being done to address the health issues and concerns of the community? What services are provided? Who participates?

- What is the cultural life of the community?

- What is being done to minimize the impact of environmental hazards on the community?

- Who are the "movers and shakers" of the community, the people who get things done and whom others in the community rely on for information and resources?

THEORETICAL CONSIDERATIONS

It is useful to conduct the community assessment using a theoretical framework because public health programs and policy initiatives are best developed using a strong theory. Examples of theoretical approaches for conducting a community assessment are available in the scientific literature. Community assessments may be based on one or a combination of individual, interpersonal, or communal theoretical models of health-behavior change. The conclusions that are drawn during the community assessment describe the relationships among the factors that cause the problem and the resources that are available.

The most commonly used theories of individual behavior in public health are the Transtheoretical Model (Procashasca & DiClemente, 1983), Social Cognitive Theory (Bandura, 1986), the Health Belief Model (Hochbaum, 1958), the Theory of Planned Behavior (Fishbain & Ajzen, 1975), and the Social Support Theory (House, 1981). At the community and group level, community organization and community building are important concepts in the absence of a single unified model (Minkler, Wallerstein, & Wilson, 2008). Table 2.1 provides an overview of the major concepts from these models; detailed descriptions can be found in Glanz, Rimer, and K. Viswanath (2008). Other theoretical frameworks have been used in public health, such as the Andersen model, which explains people's utilization of health services (Andersen, 1995).

When a theory or a theoretical framework is used for the community assessment, the same theory may be used in the development of the program. The value in using a theoretical framework for program development is that it increases the likelihood of incorporating the factors that are known to result in the change that the initiative is addressing.

THE ECOLOGICAL MODEL

Historically, behavioral theories have been the primary drivers of initiatives to address public health problems. However, recognition of the social and environmental factors that influence health has led to use of an ecological-systems perspective, which

TABLE 2.1.   **Commonly Used Theories and Models in Public Health**

Theory	Major Concepts
Transtheoretical Model Based on individuals' changing behavior through stages of readiness	Precontemplation Contemplation Preparation Action Maintenance
Social Cognitive Theory Personal factors, environmental factors, and individual behavior operate in a dynamic, reciprocal way	Reciprocal determinism Outcome expectations Self-efficacy Observational learning Self-regulation Rewards and punishments
Health Belief Model Based on individuals' perceptions of the problem and of the benefits, barriers, and factors influencing the decision to adopt a behavior	Perceived susceptibility Perceived severity Perceived benefits Perceived barriers Cues to action Self-efficacy
Theory of Planned Behavior Based on individuals' intentions, attitudes, and perceptions of social norms and their ability to perform a behavior	Behavioral intention Experiential attitude Subjective norm Perceived behavioral control
Social Support Based on individuals' perception and experience of support from those around them	Emotional support Instrumental support Informational support Appraisal support
Community Organization Hypothesizes a community-driven process for addressing health and social problems	Empowerment Critical consciousness Community capacity Social capital Issue selection Participation and relevance

incorporates in its analysis individual and environmental factors. The assessment may incorporate concepts from theoretical frameworks at each of these levels. The ecological model allows the integration of multiple theories and models as needed. It dictates that it is not sufficient to look at individual factors in a community assessment because organizational and community factors may play a role.

The ecological model may be used to provide guidance for a comprehensive approach to community assessment and program development across multiple domains of behavioral influence. At the individual level, behavior is influenced by biological, physiological, psychological, and emotional states. At the interpersonal level, structural factors and social and cultural norms of peers, family, and friends play a role. The organizational, community, and policy domains recognize the influence and impact of multiple environmental factors on behavior. Determinants at this level include economic, physical, and structural factors and systems that influence health outcomes. Where people live, work, and play significantly affects health outcomes. In addition, the social determinants of health (Commission on Social Determinants of Health, 2008) include conditions that lead to inequality and injustices that increase the risk for disease and disability and influence individual and collective health and well-being. Social cohesion, social inclusiveness, social capital, and trust are also factors in determining health outcomes (Marmot, 2004). Using the ecological model as the guiding framework allows these concepts to be included in a community assessment of factors that influence health. Incorporating core principles of the ecological model (Figure 2.3) in behavior-change models leads to behavior change through appropriate, behavior-specific interventions (Sallis, Owen, & Fisher, 2008).

FIGURE 2.3.   *The Ecological-Model Framework*

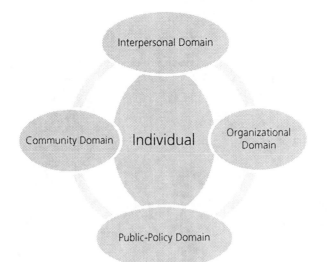

DATA COLLECTION

Data for a community assessment are collected from the population of interest to determine the incidence and prevalence rates of disease and the extent of the problem. Rates of disease and disability are described as the number of cases per 1,000 or per 100,000 of the population. In addition, risk and protective factors associated with the public health problem are identified and described. The risk factors are those personal and environment factors or determinants that increase the likelihood of an individual's coming into contact with or being exposed to conditions that lead to disease or disability. Protective factors are mirror images of risk factors; when they are present, they provide protection against the risk of or the exposure to disease or disability.

In addition to identifying risk and protective factors, a community assessment must identify human, material, and economic assets, including formal and informal community-based organizations and networks that are available in the community (Kretzmann & McKnight, 1993) to address the problem. The assessment includes demographic, social, economic, cultural, structural, and systems factors that affect the population of interest and the community. The assessment contains information about the state of the community, access to and delivery of services, cultural and social norms and practices, as well as the economic situation.

Data on the economic situation of a community include not only the educational level of the population of interest but also the types and locations of jobs that the community offers to its residents (low paying versus high paying). Such characteristics of the community's structure and systems infrastructure are an important gauge of the community's ability and willingness to support public health efforts. Determining the resources in the community identifies important allies for addressing the problem and supporting sustainable, culturally appropriate initiatives that are congruent with the reality of the community and the lives of its residents.

PROCESS

The community assessment is conducted using both qualitative and quantitative approaches (Finifter, Jensen, Wilson, & Koenig, 2005). Data are collected to understand the community's expressed and observed needs for health and social services. Carrying out a community assessment requires that the researchers follow a process that involves multiple stakeholders and uses multiple data-collection sources and methods.

Steps in conducting a community assessment include:

1. Establish a team to undertake the community assessment.

2. Determine the availability of data to assess the problem.

3. Determine which data are missing and need to be collected.

4. Decide on the data-collection approach.

5. Develop and/or secure data-collection instruments (surveys, interview guides, and so on).

6. Develop the data-collection plan.

7. Secure resources for the data-collection plan.

8. Implement the data-collection plan.

9. Analyze and interpret the data.

10. Use the information to frame the intervention.

Step 1. Establish a Team

Conducting a community assessment based on a participatory model requires equitable involvement by the community. The first step in the community assessment process is to engage those who are most affected by the problem and professionals who provide community-based services. The team consists of people who live within the community or who have an interest in the assessment being conducted. Members of the team should include those who are familiar with the problem, research methods, data-collection approaches, and data analysis. The team members' roles should be identified so each person is able to contribute to the process. Members of the community bring expertise and important perspectives with regard to the community, the population, and the risk factors associated with the problem being assessed. In the example in Table 2.2, the team comprises twelve people, half of whom are residents of the community.

The team decides on the task and specifies the aim of the community assessment: Should it be a broad assessment to determine the major problems or issues within the community or a narrow assessment of a specific problem? For example, if the problem is high rates of underage, alcohol-related motor vehicle accidents, then the team needs to understand which groups are most affected; how, when, and where the accidents occur; who might be facilitating the problem; and the best approaches for addressing the problem from the perspective of the community.

Step 2. Determine the Availability of Data

Once the aims of the community assessment have been established, the next step is to determine what information already exists. Data that are regularly collected by not-for-profit organizations and by state and local agencies should first be reviewed to determine what information is already available about the community. These data may be in multiple forms. They may be in data bases that have to be analyzed or in reports that have been compiled. The quality and the quantity of the data may be mixed and may be limited to small areas or one population group. The team must assess how useful the existing data are and whether they serve the purposes of the group. If the intent of the group is to understand the factors leading to a problem in the whole community, but a previous assessment was conducted only in the local junior college of five hundred students, it is important to collect additional data on other members of the community. Alternatively, given the example of underage drinking, data on the community may be available at the state level but

TABLE 2.2.   **The Community-Assessment Team**

Stakeholder	Contributions to the Community-Assessment Process
Project partners	Are key informants; provide insight into the public health problem and solutions; provide historical data and access to resources for data collection
Project partners	Provides feedback regarding methods and tools
Community residents (parents of children and community members)	Provide insights into the public health problem and the culture of the community; review the instruments; are key informants; survey participants; collect data
Members of the faith community, local school staff and students	Function as focus-group participants and survey participants; provide digital stories and photographs
Funders	Provide incentives for participants; cover costs of program management and data collection
Project manager and staff	Provides overall direction of community assessment; provides guidance in framing the questions; develops methodology

not give any specifics for youth. Collecting primary data from youth would then be important to support the development of the intervention. Secondary data may be available to answer some of the questions, but the team may need to collect additional data.

Using human subjects in a community assessment may require that the team has its proposal reviewed by the Institutional Review Board of the organization. Usually these boards are found in research universities. Sometimes they are called Ethics Boards.

Step 3. Determine Which Data Are Missing and Need to be Collected

After a full review of the existing data, a determination is made by the team of the additional data needs of the project. Through group consultations, a list is compiled of the information that is available and of the questions that still need to be answered. Questions may include:

- What are the problems or issues in the community, in a specific area, or with a particular group?

- How does the problem or issue affect different members of the community?

- How prevalent is the problem among members of different groups—by age, gender, race, profession, educational level, socioeconomic status, and so on?

- What are the factors that increase or decrease the occurrence of the problem?

- What are the individual, interpersonal, community, organizational, or policy factors?

- What resources—human, material, and financial—are available within the community as well as outside the community that can be brought to bear on the problem?

- Who are the people and what are the systems and structures available and ready to address the problem?

- How does addressing the problem address issues of social justice?

It is important to collect only the information that is needed and that answers the overarching research question. It is both a waste of resources and a waste of participants' time if data are collected that will not be used for program development.

Step 4. Decide on the Data-Collection Approach

The data-collection approach that is used to conduct the needs assessment takes the needs of the project into consideration. The data that are collected may be quantitative or qualitative or a combination. The most suitable data are those that provide the evidence for answering the research questions. For example, if the question to be answered is, What are the factors that influence youth drinking?, the data-collection approach can include focus groups with youth and their parents as well as other key informants like law enforcement. In addition a survey could give valuable information on the extent of the problem. The factors that determine the most appropriate approach for answering the question(s) and hence the most appropriate data to collect include the size and scope of the project, the study subject, the kind of information that is required, and the resources available for the project.

The Size and Scope of the Project   The size and scope of the project influence the data-collection approach because the larger and more spread out the population sample or the more factors being assessed, the more likely that a quantitative data method will be selected. Qualitative approaches may be used to complement quantitative approaches in large studies; in small studies qualitative approaches may be used alone. Using the ecological-model framework, which includes an assessment of factors at all levels of behavioral influence increases the size and scope of the study in innumerable ways. Increases in both the size of the sample and the scope of the project have implications for the measurement approaches that may be appropriate for assessing each dimension.

The Study Subject   The kind of subjects in the study also influences the approach used. In understanding the high rates of obesity in a community, for example, it is important to obtain information from individuals as well as to do an environmental scan of neighborhoods. In this case, the study subjects include both people and locations. Collecting data from individuals involves using surveys, individual interviews, focus groups, among other methods. The environmental scan can take on multiple forms—for example, assessing the number of fast-food restaurants or convenience stores in the neighborhood or observing the type, quantity, and quality of food that people choose to eat.

The Kind of Information Required   The kind of data that are collected is determined by the type of information that is needed. Studies of knowledge may be easily assessed using surveys, while understanding attitudes toward a behavior may be more easily assessed using focus groups. Behavior, however, may be less reliably assessed using self-reported surveys; observing the behavior provides more objective evidence. Assessing the extent to which grocery stores and farmers' markets are available within a community lends itself to using a combination of qualitative and quantitative measures. Or the kind of information required may suggest the use of photographic and digital storytelling.

The Resources Available   The financial, material, and human resources that are available for a project influence the amount of data that can be collected. The data-collection approach must also provide for the inclusion and the training of members of the community. Community members can be trained to develop the data-collection instruments and to collect and analyze the data. In general, it is critical to use the most appropriate and cost-efficient approach to collect the most useful data. It does little good to collect data using a survey because of limited resources if using a survey will not help you answer the research question.

Step 5. Develop and/or Secure Data-Collection Instruments

The questions that need to be answered as part of the community assessment will determine the data-collection instruments that are most appropriate. Using surveys allows the team to collect quantitative data and to draw conclusions about the problem using numbers (frequencies, means, univariate analysis). Other instruments allow qualitative data to be collected on perceptions, depths of feelings, experiences, attitudes, beliefs, and behaviors using qualitative approaches. These instruments can also provide information on the quality of a product or an operation, exposure to an initiative or condition, and adherence to a task or behavior.

The instrument selected will determine who should provide the data. Because data must be credible, it is important to ensure that the appropriate persons and sites are selected. Participants who experience a problem are likely to be the most credible for describing the problem, but in the assessment of assets to address the problem other people may provide different perspectives. Data obtained from multiple sources and collected using reliable tools increase the validity and the credibility of the research. Some of these tools are the following:

- Focus-group discussions are useful for obtaining information quickly and for understanding broad perspectives. Focus groups are homogenous groups of six to eight individuals who convene to answer open-ended, predetermined questions.

- Individual key-informant interviews are used to gather information from individuals who either are affected by the problem or can provide an independent perspective. Individual interviews are often carried out with opinion leaders who need to be included in the community assessment because of their unique perspectives but whose status in the community makes it preferable that they not be included in focus groups. Individual interviews are often quicker than focus groups because interviews can be scheduled more easily with one person than with six or more together.

- Photovoice is a qualitative data-collection technique in which the data are collected by members of the community using cameras. The photographs are discussed to highlight issues that the photographer identifies as relevant for describing the problem.

- Digital storytelling, which utilizes audio or video recordings, is developing into a popular approach in community needs assessments. It allows the participants to document the problem and their experiences in their own words; they can provide strong testimonials that support the development of initiatives.

- Asset maps can be used to identify and document physical or human resources within the community that may influence the problem and/or provide venues for the intervention—for example, churches, schools, health facilities, and businesses. Assets are mapped to show the quantity, distribution, and accessibility of the resources to populations of interest. A mapping of stores in low-income neighborhoods could show the number and location of food outlets compared with shops that sell alcohol. In conducting a study of the accessibility of fresh fruits and vegetables in a community that has high rates of childhood obesity, an asset map might include the availability of produce in

  - corner stores and convenience stores

  - farmers' markets

  - grocery stores

  - school vending machines

In addition, the skills, talents, and expertise of community leaders—heads of agencies, organizations, businesses, churches, schools—may be tallied to determine the level of resources available within the community for addressing the problem and developing the initiative.

Information on the instruments that can be used may be obtained by reviewing the literature and contacting others who have conducted similar studies. Surveys and other data-collection tools may also be developed for specific initiatives, although the process is time-consuming and developing a good instrument. requires a certain amount of expertise. Quantitative and qualitative data-collection methods are described in detail in Chapter Seven and Chapter Nine.

Step 6. Develop the Data-Collection Plan

A data-collection plan describes the steps that are required to ensure that the data are collected; Table 2.3 is an example of such a plan. It includes the following components:

- Data to be collected

- Methods for collecting the data

- Source of the data

- Persons responsible

A data-collection plan may also be an activity plan that outlines the time frame for data collection.

TABLE 2.3.   **Example of a Data-Collection Plan**

Data to Be Collected	Methods for Collecting the Data	Source of the Data	Person(s) Responsible
Knowledge about HIV/AIDS transmission	Existing survey developed by federally funded project	Adults eighteen to twenty-five years	Youth-development project director
Attitudes toward condoms	Focus-group discussion; interview guide developed locally	Adults eighteen to twenty-five years	Graduate assistant; project manager
Availability of condoms	Survey; observation; photography	Store owners, pharmacy managers	Project manager; leader of community-assessment team

Step 7. Secure Resources for the Data-Collection Plan

Once the team has decided on the design for the community assessment and has developed the plan, the resources for implementing the plan must be secured through grants, donations, or budgeted activities. Resources include:

- Personnel (staff and volunteers) for conducting the study

- Salaries and stipends for staff and volunteers

- Transportation

- Data-collection instruments

- Interview space

- Equipment, supplies, and materials

Step 8. Implement the Data-Collection Plan

At the implementation stage, it is assumed that all the resources are available, the materials have been developed, the study participants have been notified or recruited as required by the method, and the instruments are available and ready to use.

Let us look at an example from the data-collection plan in Table 2.3. The person responsible for ensuring that data on the availability of condoms are collected is the leader of the community-assessment team. The leader may recruit other members of the team to participate in the data collection or recruit and train others. The plan identifies the data-collection methods as surveys, observation, and photography. The survey includes items regarding the level and turnover of condom stocks in stores and pharmacies throughout the year. Observation forms and the protocol for collecting the data are developed. The protocol contains instructions for making the observation and forms for documenting the results. In addition, it contains instructions for obtaining photographs that will be helpful in making judgments about the availability and accessibility of condoms in the stores and pharmacies. Before any data are collected, the store owners and pharmacy managers are contacted to inform them of the study and the team's intention to complete a survey in order to document the availability of condoms in their stores. They are asked to provide signed consent.

Step 9. Analyze and Interpret the Data

Interpretation and analysis of data collected for a community assessment are determined by the type of data collected. Quantitative data can be analyzed manually if the sample size is small or by using computer-assisted mechanisms such as Microsoft Excel or SPSS®. Determining frequencies, means, standard deviations for the data and describing the sample is the first step. Depending on the level of data collected—ordinal, nominal, scale, or ratio data—and the sample size and questions asked, other types of analysis may be undertaken, including univariate, bivariate, and multivariate analysis. If the community assessment is made at the beginning and at the end of an intervention, a paired test may be appropriate. Graphs, charts, and maps provide a visual representation of the results.

Qualitative data is also analyzed using manual or computer-assisted approaches. Evaluating qualitative data requires content analysis to determine themes. The themes form the basis for the report and provide answers to the research questions.

The interpretation of the findings is based on the information that the community assessment set out to get and the likely use of the data. If the focus of the intervention is behavior change in the population sample, then the report may include the following:

- Frequency of the behavior

- Context of the behavior

- Environmental conditions under which the behavior is carried out

- Approaches to addressing the behavior and internal and external resources that might support the intervention

If, however, the approach is policy oriented, then the focus of the report is the information required to frame the needs for the policy and the populations or setting that the policy would need to target.

A community assessment of the physical environment could include a photovoice approach to data collection and understanding multiple perspectives.

Policy leading to social change requires a process that includes community and policymaker education, advocacy, and community mobilization and action. Understanding the requirements of the initiative for each component is critical to undertaking a meaningful policy-change process. The analysis and interpretation of the data collected during the process is based on the needs of the project. For example data may be collected to assess community mobilization and action. Data collected might include: who are mobilized, numbers, locations, and the number and type of actions that were taken as a result the mobilization. Data to analyze may range from the level of participation at events to actions taken as a result of e-mail alerts. It may also include analyzing data collected from policy makers with regards to the outcome of the actions. This data may be in multiple forms which include quantitative and qualitative formats and must be analyzed in ways appropriate for the method used.

Step 10. Use the Information to Frame the Intervention

The usual final step in the community assessment is to use the information obtained from the research to frame the new initiative. The data provide information regarding the people affected, where they live and work, the factors that predispose them to the problem, as well as those that enable or reinforce the problem. The data also includes information about the human, material and financial resources for addressing the problem.

DATA SOURCES

When community assessments are conducted, primary or secondary data may be used to assess the problem and to determine who is most affected. Primary data are collected for the purposes of the particular study, and secondary data are existing data collected for a previously defined purpose. Primary data for a community needs assessment are gathered using qualitative or quantitative approaches. It is especially important to use primary data when information about culturally diverse populations is limited and specific information is required to ensure the development of culturally appropriate interventions. Existing qualitative or quantitative data collected for other purposes may be available. Using secondary data is less time consuming and less expensive than collecting and analyzing primary data.

Primary-data collection utilizes a variety of methods, including self-administered surveys, case studies, observation, focus-group discussions, and individual interviews (Sharpe et al., 2005). Data may also be collected using face-to-face, telephone, or web-assisted technologies. Less formal assessments than these may take place when driving or walking through the community conducting an initial visual assessment, in community meetings, and when using participatory-research approaches such as photo narratives (Bender & Harbour, 2001; Sharpe et al., 2005), photovoice (Wang, Burris, & Ping, 1996), and theater, music, dance, puppet shows, and storytelling (Sharpe et al., 2005).

Large health-related assessments and existing local and state data bases in combination with census data provide valuable information for estimating the extent of a public health problem. In using secondary data it is important to check its validity, source, sample size, and nature of the sample. Other considerations in the use of secondary data include how closely the data match the public health problem being assessed and the extent to which the data reflect the local situation.

Secondary data may be obtained from death certificates; disease, disability, and crime surveillance; health records; and surveys. Useful indicators are vital statistics: births and deaths, age-specific death rates, disease-specific morbidity and mortality rates. Secondary data that may be available at state, county, and in some cases zip code level include:

- HIV/AIDS infection rates and AIDS diagnoses
- Teen pregnancy rates
- Cancer rates
- Birth and death rates
- Obesity rates
- Heart-disease rates
- Crime rates

In addition, health and wellness data may be available with indicators such as socioeconomic, environmental, and behavioral factors that influence disease risk, access to health care, and utilization of health and social services. Factors may include:

- Educational levels
- Household income levels

▓ Nature and levels of contamination of air and water

▓ Service utilization

Quality-of-life indicators such as educational attainment, employment, income, housing, safety, and human rights provide information about the public health problem and opportunities to consider holistic approaches. Census data (www.census.gov) provide demographic information for the United States down to the county level, and other community-level data may complement census data.

Applications of Geographic Information Systems mapping technologies provide a unique profile of the community by combining information from primary and secondary sources with census data (Fazlay, Lofton, Doddato, & Mangum, 2003; Harris & López-Defede, 2004). In addition, specific points of interest can be mapped using these systems to produce an asset map of the local community at zip code level.

Multiple models have been described for conducting a comprehensive community assessment, and data may be collected using a variety of tools. One example of a community assessment that is commonly used by local public health agencies is the Mobilizing for Action through Planning and Partnerships (MAPP) process (National Association of County and City Health Officials, n.d.). The tool was developed by the National Association of County and City Health Officials (NACCHO) in collaboration with the Centers for Disease Control and Prevention. The cyclical MAPP process is organized in six phases and contains four major components of the health assessment:

1. *Community themes and strengths* provides insights into issues such as perceived quality of life and the identification of assets and resources to address problems using a qualitative research approach.

2. *Local public health system assessment* assesses the structures and systems within the community that provide services and their capacities.

3. *Community health status assessment* provides quantitative data on a wide range of health indicators.

4. *Forces of change assessment* identifies forces and actions external to the health system that affect the health of the community.

(More information about this community assessment can be obtained from the NACCHO website, http://www.naccho.org/topics/infrastructure/mapp/mappbasics.cfm.)

REVIEWING THE SCIENTIFIC LITERATURE

In addition to collecting primary data and compiling secondary data, a community assessment incorporates an extensive search of the scientific literature. This review identifies known behavioral, epidemiological, social, cultural, and environmental conditions associated with the public health problem at the local, state, and national levels. It identifies current conditions and historical trends. Local and web-based library resources and a systematic search of the published research provide an opportunity to compare problems in the local community with state and national trends and to understand the

EXAMPLE

PART OF A LITERATURE REVIEW

Screening for Breast Cancer

Women who have not been screened are more likely to be diagnosed with breast cancer later than women who have been screened (Author et al., 2008). In addition, they are more likely to be older (>75 years), unmarried, with no family history of breast cancer, and with less education and lower socioeconomic status (Author, 2009).

rationale for the initiative. The literature review is focused and specific and is used to answer the following questions:

- How does the community's assessment profile compare with the profiles of other communities of similar size and demographics across the state or nationally?

- What are the most appropriate, logical, and evidence-based ways to address the problem the community identified?

Conducting a review of the literature is a systematic process that involves a number of steps, including identifying the topic and the search terms, researching the publications, and synthesizing the literature (Shi, 2008). Published peer reviewed literature is searched using traditional library or online resources such as Medline, PubMed, or ProQuest® to find relevant books, professional-journal articles, and technical reports. Peer-reviewed research is also available through advanced scholar searches using the internet search engine Google®.

For example, if the research topics are heart disease among adults and the relationship between heart disease and physical activity, the search terms may include heart disease (incidence and prevalence), heart disease and adults, heart disease and physical activity, heart disease and exercise, heart disease and gender, heart disease and risk factors (age, obesity, nutrition, race). A more refined search using these categories but with women will provide a more focused review of the literature. In addition, the search may provide insights into theories that the program may adopt to provide an understanding of the public health problem at a local, state, or national level and into the relationship between the problem and the resources and activities needed to address it.

When the search is conducted and research articles are located, the researchers review references from the previous five to ten years based on the topic and the articles' appropriateness and relevance for their work. Selected papers are reviewed closely and summarized by providing the following information: title, author, journal/book/report

FIGURE 2.4.   *Framework for Summarizing a Literature Review*

Background	• Title • Author • Journal year, volume, issue, page number	
Design	• Descriptive, quazi-experimental, experimental • Reseach, evaluation • Population/sample size • Research question	
Research and Results	• Research methods and approaches • Variables included • Data analysis • Results and significant findings	

publication information, the study or intervention design (type of intervention or type of study, population or sample size, and so on). In addition, the summary contains the research question, the variables, the data-analysis approach and statistical methods, the results of the study, and significant findings. Issues of reliability and validity are also noted. Figure 2.4 provides a framework for summarizing a literature review.

When the search is complete and there are enough articles to provide a sufficiently detailed background to the problem and its potential solutions, the literature review is written. The literature review is a synthesis of all the papers reviewed with regard to a specific research question. The synthesis consists of "analyzing and interpreting [the article's] findings and summarizing those findings into unified statements about the topic being reviewed" (Shi, 2008, p. 117). The literature review may be organized under appropriate headings to capture the overall theme of a paragraph, and each paragraph must be linked to the previous paragraph by a suitable transition. The review of the scientific literature is a component of the community-assessment report and later will form part of the introduction and background section of the evaluation report.

THE REPORT

The community-assessment report is a summary of the results of the assessment and the review of the scientific literature. It is a discussion of priorities for addressing the public health problem in a considered and logical way. The results of the quantitative-data analysis are shown in narrative form as well as in charts, tables, and graphs to ensure easy understanding. Qualitative data are summarized, and samples of the data are presented as quotations to allow the reader to make independent interpretations. The easier the report is to follow, the more likely it is to be used. The report outlines the research approach, the results, and discussions of the results and their implications. An outline of the components of an assessment report is provided here.

Literature-Review Section

The literature review describes the public health problem(s) being investigated from the perspective of the existing literature:

▓   The rates of disease or disability (number of cases per 1,000 or 100,000 population) in the community compared with state and national rates

▓   Trends in the prevalence and incidence of disease and disability in the community compared with state and national trends

▓   The social, economic, and cultural environment that drives the problem/condition

▓   Risk and protective factors associated with the problem as seen in state and national data

▓   Peer, family, community, institutional, policy, structural, and systems influences associated with the problem

Methodology and Results Section

This section describes the methodology used for the community assessment:

▓   The sample characteristics (primary data and secondary data)

▓   The data-collection approach

▓   The data analysis

This section also discusses the results of the community assessment. It organizes the results of the analysis in a systematic way. The results may be organized in order by answering each research question or by using the theoretical framework that was used to design the study. Alternatively the results may be organized to describe

▓   the extent of the public health problem(s) of the population and of population segments by age, gender, life stage, and ethnicity (if appropriate)

▓   risk and protective factors associated with the public health problem

▓   peer, family, and community influences associated with the problem

▓   community, institutional, public-policy, structural, and systems factors that influence the problem

In addition, this section describes the human, material, and economic assets available in the community to address the problem:

▓   Individual knowledge, skills, and resources of community members, agency personnel, and others

▓ Interpersonal actions and norms

▓ Existing community resources and services

▓ Institutional resources (financial and material)

▓ Resources for developing public policy

In addition, this section suggests potential community-based, culturally appropriate ways to address the problem in the most comprehensive way. And, finally, it discusses limitations that may have resulted in bias in the study and in the conclusions—for example, small sample size, inappropriateness of the instrument, loss of study participants. Such issues may affect the researcher's confidence in the results.

STAKEHOLDERS' PARTICIPATION IN COMMUNITY ASSESSMENTS

There are multiple opportunities for stakeholders to participate in a community assessment. Consistent with the Participatory Model for Evaluation described in this book, identifying and engaging stakeholders occurs in the first step. Representatives of all stakeholder groups should be involved in the community-assessment process from the start so that they have a sense of ownership in both the process and the product. Including a mapping of community assets in the process allows stakeholders to identify and mobilize existing community resources to address community problems (Sharpe et al., 2005).

Stakeholders can have one or more roles in the process. They may initiate and conduct the community assessment or serve as participants in the study. Stakeholder involvement may include designing the study, the data-collection methodology, and the instrument(s) as well as collecting or providing the data. Some stakeholders may not be directly connected with the program, but they can provide valuable perspectives. Savage and colleagues involved stakeholders as key informants in the analysis of emerging themes during their research (Savage, Xu, Lee, Rose, Kappesser, & Anthony, 2006). Some stakeholders are intimately connected to the problem, and they are able to bring the core values and unique culture of the population of interest into focus. They have insight into how they experience the problem, the risk and protective factors, as well as community, institutional, and policy structures that influence the public health problem.

An important stakeholder group that emerged in the early years of the HIV/AIDS epidemic was those who were infected and affected by HIV/AIDS. They became important advocates for their own needs and important partners in the fight against the spread of HIV and the provision of treatment for those infected. They are contributors to the process, providing guidance and resources in addition to being participants in research.

Stakeholder participation is critical for ensuring that the sample population is knowledgeable about the study and is willing to participate. In small and rural communities previous knowledge of a research activity often facilitates data collection and ensures there is appropriately obtained informed consent. Information about impending community assessments can be provided in community meetings and in print and electronic media. It is important that the potential study respondents understand the value of participating in the study to ensure valid and reliable information to inform decision making.

SUMMARY

▓ Public health program and policy initiatives are developed in response to a public health concern when individuals, organizations, or agencies identify a problem to be addressed.

▓ Conducting a thorough community assessment that includes both needs and assets ensures the identification and development of suitable approaches for addressing the problem.

▓ The community assessment is part of a cyclical and iterative process; it precedes the initiative's implementation and/or follows the initiative's evaluation.

▓ Using a participatory approach by including community members and those who are most closely associated with the problem ensures program development and implementation that are both culturally appropriate and sustainable.

▓ Community assessments include factors that influence health at the individual, interpersonal, community, institutional, and public-policy levels.

▓ Data for a community assessment may be primary or secondary data collected using qualitative or quantitative approaches.

▓ Reviewing the scientific literature provides a broad perspective of the problem of who are affected; of why, how, and when they were affected. It also provides guidance for influencing the problem.

DISCUSSION QUESTIONS AND ACTIVITIES

1. Define *community assessment*. Provide an example of community assessment and draw a graph, picture, or in other ways illustrate what the term means to you.

2. Select a public health problem and conduct a literature review focusing on the epidemiological and behavioral data. Identify the risk factors that influence the problem. Write a three-page summary of your findings.

3. Conduct a literature search and find at least two articles in which the author has described how a needs or community assessment was conducted. What theoretical framework was used, and what research approaches were applied?

KEY TERMS

community assessment
community organization
ecological model
Health Belief Model
literature review
MAPP
primary data
risk factors

secondary data
Social Cognitive Theory
Social Support Theory
Theory of Planned Behavior
Transtheoretical Model
stakeholders
theory

3

DEVELOPING INITIATIVES

AN OVERVIEW

LEARNING OBJECTIVES

- Identify and describe the elements in program planning and implementation.
- Explain how objectives are used in program planning.
- Describe a program's Theory of Change.
- Develop a logic model.
- Explain the role of stakeholders in program implementation.

Program development and implementation is the process through which people, conditions, and environments are changed to improve population health outcomes. Although priorities for intervening with programs or policy initiatives are identified during the community assessment, guidance for focusing the initiative and identifying targets for the intervention may be found in lists of national or international goals and objectives. Healthy People 2010 (U.S. Department of Health and Human Services. 2000) specifies two overarching health goals for the United States and identifies ten leading health indicators.

The two goals of Healthy People 2010 are increasing the quality and years of healthy life and eliminating health disparities. Ten important public health goals were identified as the bases for developing programs and policy:

1. Increasing physical activity

2. Reducing the rates of obesity

3. Reducing the morbidity and mortality associated with tobacco use

4. Reducing the morbidity and mortality associated with substance abuse

5. Reducing the rates of sexually transmitted diseases

6. Maintaining mental health

7. Reducing the rates of injury and violence

8. Improving air quality

9. Increasing immunization rates

10. Increasing access to health care

(A full list of the Healthy People 2010 objectives may be found at http://www.healthy-people.gov/.)

The Millennium Development Goals 2015 (United Nations, 2008) lists eight international goals with development targets for 2015:

1. Eradicate extreme poverty and hunger

2. Achieve universal primary education

3. Promote gender equity and empower women

4. Reduce child mortality

5. Improve maternal health

6. Combat HIV/AIDS, malaria, and other diseases

7. Ensure environmental sustainability

8. Develop a global partnership for development

(The 2008 report can be found at http://www.un.org/millenniumgoals/pdf/The%20Millennium%20Development%20Goals%20Report%202008.pdf.)

Selection of the program and policy initiatives to be implemented is influenced by multiple factors that reflect the organization's overall mission. The organization's mission provides the direction for program planning and implementation. In a hypothetical example, high rates of diabetes in a community led to the development of an initiative to prevent the onset of diabetes in those at risk of the disease. The community assessment found that those most likely to have diabetes were black and female and had not completed high school. In addition, it found that among those between the ages of forty-five and sixty-four the number of new cases of diabetes was 6.9 per 1,000, a significant increase from that of the eighteen to forty-four year olds, whose rate was 2 per 1,000. Rates were even higher among those sixty-five and older. An additional finding was that women were more likely to be obese than men. The community decided to tackle the problem by developing a diabetes-prevention initiative.

Embedded within this information are a number of facts that would influence one or more organizations to develop program or policy initiatives. The organizations most likely to take on the task of reducing the rates of diabetes in the population would likely have missions that encompass this population group and would have the capacity to effect change. This chapter discusses the development of public health interventions as a prelude to program evaluation.

THE ORGANIZATION'S MISSION

The mission of an organization is reflected in its mission statement and mirrors the organization's charge, direction, and population focus. It is the foundation for the planning process and the development of goals, objectives, and activities to address the public health problem.

The mission statement announces the public health problem that the organization wishes to address in the broadest perspective. A strong mission statement for an organization contains the following components:

▓ The desired outcome of its programs

▓ The population that will be the target of its work

▓ The geographical community it serves

An example of an organization's mission statement could be to "improve the quality of lives of African American women in Riverside County." Another organization's mission could be to "reduce the rates of chronic disease among women who live in the state." Both organizations could use their missions to address the high rates of diabetes among black, low-income females. However, each organization might take a different approach to achieving the same goal. For example, one organization might chose to provide increased access to health care to improve treatment opportunities for those with diabetes; the other organization might focus on prevention of the onset of diabetes. Irrespective of the approach that is taken, the next steps in the process are planning and implementing the initiative.

PLANNING THE INITIATIVE

Building Community Support

The social, political, and cultural environment of the community provides a context for the organization's programs and policy initiatives. These factors determine the types of programs that the organization offers, its funding level, and community support for its initiatives. Community support influences initiative development and implementation in many ways.

When a community-based organization or an agency identifies a problem and develops a program, its ability to sustain the program is often influenced by social, political, and cultural factors in the community. Social and political factors influence people's attitudes toward population groups and causes.

When support for addressing the problem is high, programs are able to attract attention from many sectors, obtain adequate funding for program development, and recruit participants. However, when support is low, the organization may have difficulty securing sufficient funding, and members of the community may not use its services or participate in its activities. Good examples of initiatives whose development is often limited because of low community support (probably based on a combination of social and political factors) are providing community-based care for people with behavioral disabilities and providing shelter for the homeless.

Community support provides evidence for potential funders that the program is well accepted by the community. It ensures the credibility of the organization and demonstrates that community members believe that the initiative is making a difference. In addition, community support is critical for the development of coalitions to provide programs and policies. Conversely, a lack of support from key individuals, organizations, or sectors of the community works against the organization and influences the public's perception of an issue and the organization's approaches. It is therefore important to solicit the support of influential community members, other organizations that do similar or complementary work, people who are directly affected by the issue, and organizations and agencies that provide a voice for the community such as advocates and media outlets. Political leaders are also important stakeholders in the development of programs and the funding of initiatives.

A well-designed initiative developed to address a particular public health issue uses community and epidemiological data to guide the development of goals and objectives, which are achieved through evidence-based and theoretically sound activities supported by strong administrative capacity.

Providing Administrative Capacity

Strong administrative capacity is important for developing and delivering quality programs. Administrative capacity influences the type of programs and the size and scope of program activities. Administrative capacity for program delivery includes having physical structures, oversight, and staffing to ensure adequate and appropriate program implementation. Administrative capacity thus includes:

- The physical structures that house the initiative components

- Managers, including board members, staff, outreach personnel, and volunteers

- Program operations and activities for each initiative

- Equipment and supplies suitable for program implementation

- Ability to address challenges posed by the initiative

Using Community Assessment and Epidemiological Data

The community assessment and epidemiological data are used in determining the direction of the public health program or policy initiative. They provide a fact-based rationale for the intervention and define the populations that, if targeted for the intervention, would benefit most. Furthermore, data that are used at the start of the program can form the baseline against which the proposed intervention outcomes can be assessed later.

Community assessment and epidemiological data contained within reports and the literature review provide information that is helpful for developing a detailed plan for the initiative. This information includes:

- The health problem, prevalence and incidence of disease, and quality-of-life indicators

- Risk and protective factors that influence the behavior of individuals

- Sociocultural and political factors that reinforce or enable conditions that increase the public health problem

- Assets and resources available within the community

GOALS AND OBJECTIVES

Developing sound initiatives requires developing goals and objectives. Unlike the mission statement, which is broad, *goals* provide clear direction, and *objectives* provide specific benchmarks for the initiative (see Figure 3.1). Objectives serve as the benchmarks for determining the level of implementation of the initiative and its outcomes. As mentioned above, the Healthy People 2010 (U.S. Department of Health and Human Services, 2000) and the Millennium 2015 (United Nations, 2008) documents provide guidance for identifying specific targets of the intervention. Going back to our previous example of diabetes, we note that HP 2010 has seventeen diabetes-related objectives. Each can be used to develop activities, and together they form the initiative to address the problem.

The Initiative (Public Health) Goal

The initiative's goal closely matches the mission of the organization and relates to the particular public health problem that is being addressed. The goal provides the initiative's direction and is a stated desire to meet an expressed and unmet population need. It is made up of three elements:

1. Describes who will be affected by the program or policy initiative

2. Communicates the intentions of the program

3. Specifies broad changes that will occur as a result of the initiative

If the mission of the organization is to "improve the health of women who live in the state," then the goal of the initiative may be to "reduce the rates of diabetes among and improve the quality of life for low-income African American women in Riverside County." In analyzing this goal we realize it contains all the components of a goal, as shown in Table 3.1.

FIGURE 3.1.   *The Hierarchical Relationship of Goals and Objectives*

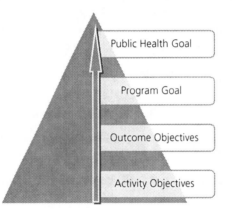

TABLE 3.1.   Goal Analysis

Goal: Reduce the rates of diabetes among and improve the quality of life for low-income African American women in Riverside County.	
Describes who will be affected by the program or policy initiative	Low-income African American women in Riverside County
Communicates the intentions of the program	To develop prevention or policy initiatives that target the risk and protective factors that influence rates of diabetes
Specifies broad changes that will occur as a result of the initiative	Reduced rates of diabetes and improved quality of life

Program Goal

The program goal reflects the initiative goal but is written to be more specific. The program/health goal identifies

- who benefits from the program
- the health benefits they will receive
- when the benefits will be achieved

For example, if the program goal is to "reduce the proportion of low-income African American women who get diabetes by 2020 from 30 percent to 10 percent," the people who benefit are low-income African American women; they receive as a benefit a reduction in the incidence of diabetes from 30 percent to 10 percent; and this benefit will be achieved by 2020.

Initiative Objectives

The initiative objectives are developed to support the program goal. The objectives outline the initiative's precise direction and define its planned purposes. Objectives provide

- small steps (benchmarks) that if completed will achieve the goal; they define specifically the road to success
- part of the blueprint for program replication
- short-, medium-, or long-term benchmarks of the program's implementation
- guidance for developing activities
- guidance for program evaluation

Because the objectives are an important aspect of the evaluation, as they are used to specify its focus, they must be consistent with the organization's mission and the initiative goal, and they must be realizable during the life and the funding of the program.

Well-developed objectives are defined as being specific, measurable, appropriate, realistic, and achievable in a specified time frame. A useful acronym for developing objectives and remembering their attributes is SMART. Let us consider what each of these terms mean.

- *Specific:* Does the objective clearly specify what will be accomplished?
- *Measurable:* Are the changes that are specified to occur measurable in appropriate and culturally sensitive ways?
- *Appropriate:* Do the changes that are to occur for the participant or in the environment make sense given what the intervention is trying to accomplish?
- *Realistic:* Are the changes achievable given the time frame, the population, the resources, and the experience of the organization?
- *Timed:* Is the time frame for accomplishing the changes specified and realistic?

Table 3.2 is an example of the application of the SMART attributes to an objective. There are two kinds of initiative objectives: outcome objectives and activity objectives.

Outcome Objectives Outcome objectives are written to guide the achievement of a program goal. They are important for assessing progress and the ultimate success of the initiative.

A *specific* outcome objective indicates what is going to change and by how much it is going to change. We can learn a number of things from the following hypothetical objective: "increase the proportion of low-income African American women who consume five portions of fruits and vegetables a day from 30 percent to 60 percent by 2012." First, we learn that the program developers intend to provide an intervention that will result in participants increasing their consumption of fruits and vegetables. Second, we learn that they expect that the proportion of women in their program who

TABLE 3.2. Applying the SMART Attributes

Objective: Reduce the proportion of low-income African American women in the program who get diabetes from 30 percent to 10 percent by 2020.	
Specific: Does the objective clearly specify what will be accomplished?	Yes. The objective is a reduction in the proportion of low-income African American women in the program who get diabetes from 30 percent to 10 percent.
Measurable: Are the changes that are specified to occur measurable in appropriate and culturally sensitive ways?	Yes. Diabetes can be diagnosed using approaches that are culturally sensitive.
Appropriate: Do the changes that are to occur for the participant or in the environment make sense given what the intervention is trying to accomplish?	Yes. The changes that will occur for the women through the program will reduce their risk of progressing to diabetes.
Realistic: Are the changes achievable given the time frame, the population, the resources, and the experience of the organization?	Yes. Improved nutrition and regular exercise have been shown to improve health; the organization has the resources and experience to provide adequate programs.
Timed: Is the time frame for accomplishing the changes specified and realistic?	Yes. Setting the year 2020 as the end point is realistic given the changes that need to occur.

increase their consumption of fruits and vegetables will increase to 60 percent. Third, we learn that the baseline that the program is using, against which they will assess their progress, is a current proportion of 30 percent; in other words, nearly one in three low-income African American women eats fewer than five portions of fruits and vegetables a day without an intervention. In general, a specific objective contains the expected outcome against which the effectiveness of the organization will be measured. In this case, the expected outcome is that women who participate in the intervention will consume five portions of fruits and vegetables a day by 2012. This provides an intermediate benchmark to reducing the proportion of women who get diabetes by 2020.

The objectives set the stage for the level of intensity of the program. The intensity of the program determines the likelihood of its being able to accomplish the goals and objectives, so the higher the target the more intense the program needs to be. In the example above, if the program is of low intensity, the initiative may get the rate down to only 20 percent rather than 10 percent. To give another example, an education intervention that only provides information to change knowledge is likely to do that fairly easily, so expecting 90 percent of the participants to increase their knowledge of, let us say, methods of HIV/AIDS transmission is realistic even after a three-hour session. This objective could read, "By the end of the training 90 percent of participants will explain all the methods of HIV/AIDS transmission." However, specifying a change in behavior with regard to preventing HIV infection would require a more intense intervention for a longer time and with a lower likelihood of success, so the target would be lower. Such an objective will be appropriately stated as, "By the end of the year, 60 percent of program participants will use condoms consistently."

Behavior change to improve health outcomes is influenced by multiple risk factors. These are the characteristics that we attempt to modify in order to achieve the behavior change. These factors occur in the individual and in the environment in which the individual lives, works, and plays.

Individual level—intellectual ability, beliefs, values, skills, maturity, and health

Interpersonal level—the relationships an individual has with family, peers, significant others

Organizational level—the resources, support, goods, and services provided by an organization or institution

Community level—societal norms, social networks, social capital, access to goods and services

Public-policy level—laws and regulations that support or discourage healthy behaviors and access to goods and services

Changes in risk factors may include increasing knowledge, changing peer norms, and improving physical structures to increase the likelihood of eating in a healthy way or of exercising. Changes in behavior may include increasing physical activity, eating healthier foods, obtaining health care, enacting health policy.

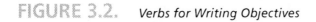

FIGURE 3.2. *Verbs for Writing Objectives*

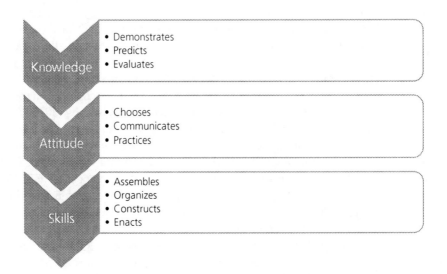

To be *measurable,* outcome objectives should incorporate verbs that are action oriented and can be assessed using available measurement tools (Figure 3.2 provides examples of action-oriented verbs). Outcomes are measured using surveys, observation, interviews, photography, and so forth. Verbs such as *understand* and *appreciate* are difficult to measure using such tools.

Writing a specific, measurable outcome objective goes hand-in-hand with writing a *realistic* objective that has a *specified time frame,* the time it should take to accomplish the objective. Time lines reflect a progression from achieving objectives easily to achieving them with difficulty. For example, changing knowledge is fairly simple and can often be done in a single session, but changing behavior or enacting legislation may take many and varied activities and great effort to accomplish.

Objectives are short, medium, and long term. Consider a time frame of ten years. Short-term objectives would fall within the first one to two years; intermediate objectives, between two and five years; and long-term objectives, between six and ten years.

Objectives that focus on the individual level and on knowledge gain as the outcome are generally short term and limited in reaching overall goals. Skill-building objectives are generally short to medium term, and behavior-change objectives are medium to long term. Objectives at the interpersonal, organizational, or community level may also have different periods of time depending on the outcome expected. For example, changing community norms or improving access to resources may require short-, medium-, and long-term outcome objectives that provide benchmarks for change over an extended period. Policy outcome objectives are usually written for the longest time frames because they require a considerable amount of effort. Changing

TABLE 3.3. **Writing Time Lines into Objectives**

Type of Change Required	Time Frame for Change	Objective
Policy	Short term	By 2012 90 percent of coalition members will know how to contact their legislators.
	Medium term	By 2013 50 percent of coalition members will take at least one action per month in support of legislation for children to have thirty minutes of exercise during the school day.
	Long term	By 2015 state legislation will be enacted to ensure that children in all fifty counties get at least thirty minutes of exercise during the school day.
Individual	Short term	By 2012 90 percent of women will know the importance of having a mammogram for the early detection of breast cancer.
	Long term	By 2015 90 percent of women over the age of forty will have a mammogram once a year.

policy first requires increasing knowledge and understanding of the need for the policy. This first step leads to the development of coalitions and advocacy. The actions of coalitions lead to procedures for the development or change of a policy. Only after these steps is the policy enacted. The time it takes to enact a policy will depend on the type of policy, the level at which it is enacted (local, state, or national), and the political climate. Table 3.3 demonstrates how to write time lines into objectives.

In adopting the ecological model for addressing a public health problem, an organization chooses to develop initiatives at multiple levels. The more levels that are included in the initiative, the more likely the health problem will be addressed from a holistic perspective and take into account not only individual factors but also, for example, peer influences on community norms and services, organizational structure and functioning, and local or national public policy.

Activity Objectives   There are a small number of outcome objectives, but there are many activity objectives that are directed toward achieving each outcome objective.

The activity objectives specify the activities for carrying out the initiative. Together the objectives and the activities are the blueprint for replication of the initiative. Ultimately, it is the activities in the initiative that result in the outcomes specified.

Activity objectives are the most frequently written objectives and the most familiar. They specify organizational and administrative tasks. They guide the implementation of the initiative and become the process objectives in the evaluation. They are used to monitor and evaluate the initiative's level of implementation and progress.

Activity objectives should answer the following questions:

- What activity will be carried out to support the outcome objective?

- Who will conduct the activity?

- When will the activity be carried out?

- Where will the activity occur?

THE INITIATIVE ACTIVITIES

The initiative activities are the best approaches for achieving the objectives. For example, it is well recognized that to reduce obesity, both healthy eating and exercise are required; so initiatives and their activities are developed to address both. Activities are based on a number of factors, including the demographic characteristics of the

EXAMPLE

ACTIVITY OBJECTIVES

1. Fitness staff will conduct a three-day interactive educational and skill-building workshop starting on day 1 of the Regent Gym Cycling intervention in the gymnasium.

2. Thirty women forty to sixty years old will participate in the ninety-day Regent Gym Cycling intervention in the gymnasium.

3. Women forty to sixty years old will identify a buddy to walk with for forty-five minutes each day.

4. Volunteers from the Regent Gym will provide information and outreach activities in the community surrounding the Regent Gym for sixty days before the start of the Regent Gym Cycling intervention to raise awareness of the importance of exercise for cardiac health.

beneficiaries of the initiative; the risk and protective factors involved; the human, financial, and material resources available. The most appropriate approaches for achieving an outcome are identified from

* conducting a review of the research literature
* identifying theory-driven programs that address the same or similar issues
* identifying evidence-based best-practice models
* consulting with local, state, and national organizations and experts doing similar work

The activities must be appropriate for achieving the objective. For example, if the objective is to improve the skills of young people to perform a certain task, then the activities that are identified must provide skill-building opportunities so that the youth learn and then practice the skill to proficiency. Likewise, if the outcome objective is to enact a policy, then the activities that are undertaken must clearly and logically lead to involvement and actions by policymakers. Activities to change policy may include:

* Education to change knowledge, beliefs, and attitudes
* Advocacy to increase understanding and relevance
* Media communications to expand the reach of the message and to change public opinion and perceptions
* Message development to target the message for particular groups
* Training to develop a cadre of advocates, message champions, and new leaders
* Outreach to increase the volunteer core
* Meetings with policymakers to facilitate increased ownership of the issue
* Development of information sheets and briefs
* Building the capacity of the organization to handle the work (increasing staff, technology, infrastructure, staff development)

Overall, appropriate activities have the following characteristics:

* They are likely to lead to the change that is specified in the objective.
* They can be completed during the specified time frame.
* They are conducted by an organization that has sufficient resources and personnel.
* They are appropriate given the culture and expectations of the population for whom they are intended.
* They form part of an overall plan to achieve a program's goal.

Activities should preferably be based on established public health theory-based approaches that have been shown to have an effect on risk and protective factors. Any theories that have been used as part of the community assessment should be used to frame the activities. See Glanz, Rimer, and Viswanath (2008) for a detailed explanation of the use of theory. The theories most often used in public health are summarized in Glanz and National Cancer Institute (U.S.) (2005). There is a greater likelihood of incorporating all the factors that are known to result in a given change if the activities are based on theoretical constructs than if they are not.

USING EXISTING EVIDENCE-BASED PROGRAMS

An alternative to developing initiatives from scratch is to identify and adopt already tested evidence-based programs that have proven to be effective (Figure 3.3). An evidence-based program is based on the most rigorous scientific evidence through a well-designed intervention-research study that is often supported by both qualitative and quantitative data. The evidence-based initiative selected for adoption should relate to the needs of the project and have similar goals and objectives.

Certain characteristics are associated with evidence-based initiatives:

▦ They specify the population that the intervention was tested with.

▦ They are based on research conducted using experimental or quasi-experimental designs with control groups.

▦ They identify the specific effects of the intervention on those who received the intervention compared with those who were in the control group.

▦ They provide sufficient information for replication.

FIGURE 3.3. *Components of Evidence-Based Programs*

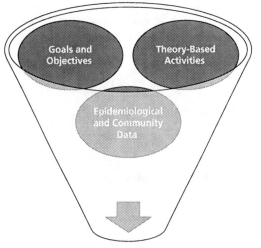

Evidence-Based Programs

Evidence-based interventions are now recommended in clinical and prevention programs in medicine, social work, and public health. For example, the Substance Abuse and Mental Health Services Association hosts the National Registry of Evidence-Based Programs and Practices, which contains a searchable data base of 137 substance-abuse and mental-health-related interventions (Substance Abuse and Mental Health Administration, 2008).

The Centers for Disease Control and Prevention developed the Tiers of Evidence conceptual framework (Centers for Disease Control and Prevention, 2007), which provides a system for classifying behavioral interventions based on the level of evidence for reducing the risk of HIV (Figure 3.4). The system has four distinct tiers: Tier 1 and Tier II interventions are those classified as evidence based. Tier III and Tier IV consist of behavioral-theory-based interventions. The system is based on the quality and rigor of the studies of an intervention and the strength of the findings. Tier I interventions are the most vigorously evaluated, while Tier IV includes programs with the least amount of empirical evidence. (Additional information about the Tiers of Evidence system can be found at http://www.cdc.gov/hiv/topics/research/prs/print/tiers-of-evidence.htm.)

Sources of information regarding evidence-based and theory-based programs and principles that reduce the risk of a disease or disability include:

▓ Published articles and reports available on the internet or in libraries

▓ Reports from or consultation with local, state, national, and international organizations

▓ Independent private and public research institutions

▓ Public health practitioners

It is important to think critically about adopting evidence-based interventions because they may have been developed for a population different from your own. Questions to consider in determining whether an existing program can be adopted for your population:

▓ What changes does the program target? Are these the same as those for the intervention being considered?

FIGURE 3.4.   *Classification System for Evidence-Based HIV/AIDS Interventions*

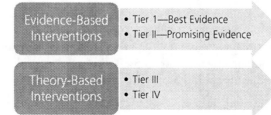

▓ Does the intervention serve a population with the same or similar characteristics?

▓ Are the appropriate resources available to implement the initiative?

▓ Can the initiative be implemented as described by the developers of the intervention?

▓ Are the intervention activities and delivery mechanisms culturally appropriate?

THE PROGRAM'S THEORY OF CHANGE

Irrespective of the approach used for developing the initiative, it is important to demonstrate a clear and logical relationship among the mission, goals, objectives, and activities in the program's Theory of Change, its operational theory. The Theory of Change is the theoretical foundation of the initiative. It explains what the organization is hoping to achieve with the initiative, the rationale for the program, and the program's goals, objectives, and activities. It describes how the resources and activities lead to attaining initiative objectives and goals. It is best developed by working with the stakeholders. Kirkhart (2005) cautions that it is important to consider the cultural context of the initiative and how it is represented in the theoretical perspectives.

THE LOGIC MODEL DEPICTING THE THEORY OF CHANGE

The logic model is a graphic or pictorial depiction of a program's Theory of Change (Frechtling, 2007). The only requirement for a logic model is that it tell the story of the intervention in a condensed and understandable format. A detailed discussion of logic models is provided in Frechtling (2007).

A logic model is

▓ a way to map a program during the planning or evaluation phase

▓ a way to show the program developers' chain of reasoning and to provide a process for understanding the program's activities and how they link to the outcomes

▓ a tool to facilitate stakeholder insight and reflection

▓ a tool to inform monitoring and the development of benchmarks to focus the evaluation

▓ a tool to help others understand the thinking of the program developers

An alternative use of the logic model may be in managing the project through a depiction of the activities and their implementation.

Components

A logic model shows diagrammatically the initiative's basic components: resources, activities, outputs, and outcomes (Figure 3.5). To keep the purpose of the program in full view, the public health goal, the program goal, and the outcome objectives are

FIGURE 3.5.   *Basic Framework for a Logic Model*

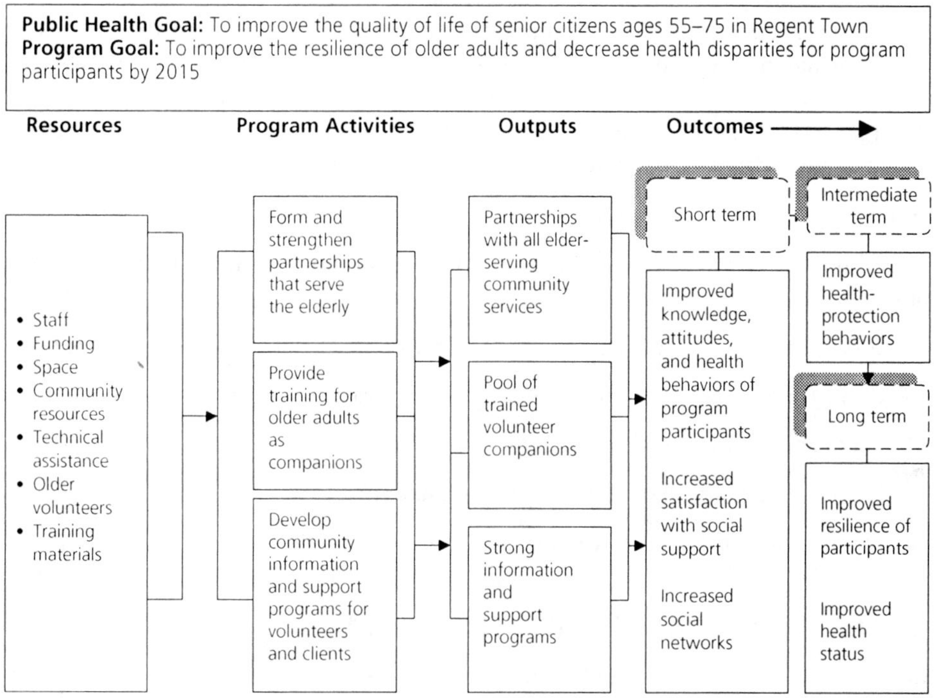

Public Health Goal: To improve the quality of life of senior citizens ages 55–75 in Regent Town
Program Goal: To improve the resilience of older adults and decrease health disparities for program participants by 2015

Resources	Program Activities	Outputs	Outcomes ⟶

Resources	Program Activities	Outputs	Short term / Intermediate term / Long term
• Staff • Funding • Space • Community resources • Technical assistance • Older volunteers • Training materials	Form and strengthen partnerships that serve the elderly	Partnerships with all elder-serving community services	**Intermediate term**
	Provide training for older adults as companions	Pool of trained volunteer companions	Improved health-protection behaviors
	Develop community information and support programs for volunteers and clients	Strong information and support programs	**Long term** Improved resilience of participants Improved health status

Outcomes (Short term): Improved knowledge, attitudes, and health behaviors of program participants; Increased satisfaction with social support; Increased social networks

noted at the top of the logic model. In addition the logic model identifies the points at which the process evaluation activities are important.

A logic model needs to include the following components:

Resources (sometimes called the *inputs*): The human, financial, and material resources that are used for the initiative. They include staff and other personnel who will be available to work on the program, grant and other monies allocated for the program, as well as office space, training materials, and other resources that are provided for the initiative.

Program activities: The specific activities that participants take part in or are exposed to that will result in changes in the participants. Examples of activities are workshops, training, educational outreach programs, coalition building, policy framing, and advocacy.

Outputs: The initial products of the initiative, the results of the intervention. Examples of outputs are the number of people trained, the number of pieces of material distributed, the number of media spots provided, the number of legislative drafts written.

Outcomes: Changes that occur in the participants in the program or those who are exposed to the policy. Outcomes may be developed as short term, intermediate term, and long term during the planning process. Examples of outcomes are an increase in knowledge, a change in attitudes, a change in behavior, increasing social support and social networks, passing a policy or legislation.

Program goal: Based on the public health goal but focused on the population served by the initiative. It provides the specific direction for the program.

Public health goal: The impact of the combined efforts of all the initiatives of all the organizations in the community that work to achieve a common goal. It expresses the expected improvement in the quality of life of the community's residents.

Criteria

A well-developed logic model may be used as a tool throughout the iterative process of program planning and is useful if it

- is detailed yet not overwhelming and contains crucial elements of the intervention
- clearly shows the relationships among the program inputs, outputs, and outcomes
- is understood by the stakeholders
- is complementary to other management materials

Note than an initiative may have more than one logic model.

CRITERIA FOR SUCCESSFUL INITIATIVES

In order to solve public health problems, initiatives for tackling them must be effective. Successful initiatives have the following criteria:

- They are comprehensive and address multiple risk factors and the social determinants of health while recognizing and strengthening protective factors.
- They address the needs of the population specifically and are culturally sensitive and appropriate.
- They are sustained over a long period.
- They address problems that concern the community, which supports finding solutions.
- They have well-trained, managed staff.
- They are well resourced.

  Effective programs have the following characteristics:

- Activities are appropriate for accomplishing the objectives.
- Human, material, and financial resources are adequate.
- Activities reflect cultural sensitivity.
- Staff are trained and adequately prepared to deliver/support the initiative.

▨   A clearly articulated time line for implementing the initiative is followed.

▨   Barriers to program implementation are recognized and solutions are identified.

▨   Effective strategies to market the program and recruit participants are utilized.

▨   Monitoring and evaluation data-collection tools are developed and utilized to assess program implementation and outcomes,

In addition, developing appropriate and effective initiatives to address public health problems requires input from a range of stakeholders. A critical stakeholder in the initiation of the program or policy initiative is the funder. The funder provides the resources for the program and oversight, often as a member of the board of directors. Other stakeholders include those who provide oversight and those who will benefit from the program.

The development of culturally appropriate and sustainable programs that lead to empowerment (Rappaport, 1984) requires the establishment of effective partnerships with all stakeholders (Panet-Raymond, 1992). The partnerships are strengthened by the participation of stakeholders in multiple tasks, including:

▨   Reviewing the community assessment

▨   Developing the mission, goals, and objectives

▨   Identifying appropriate theories, theory-based initiatives, and evidence-based programs

▨   Identifying activities for program implementation

▨   Designing a program and developing the program's Theory of Change

▨   Identifying resources (human, financial, and material) for program implementation

▨   Initiating and overseeing program implementation

▨   Developing an evaluation plan and identifying an evaluator

SUMMARY

▨   The mission statement reflects the organization's mission, direction, and population focus.

▨   The initiative is developed based on the findings of the community assessment; the mission; and the social, political, and cultural contexts in which the program operates.

▨   Outcome objectives provide benchmarks for achievement of the program goal. Outcome objectives frame the initiative in multiple domains—individual, interpersonal, organizational, community, and public-policy.

▨   Well-developed outcome and activity objectives serve as tools in the evaluation.

(Continued)

(Continued)

▩   Initiatives include theory-based or evidence-based programs.

▩   Logic models depict the Theory of Change of an initiative in graphic or pictorial terms. The logic model informs the monitoring of the initiative and focuses the evaluation. Components of the logic model are resources, activities, outputs, and outcomes.

DISCUSSION QUESTIONS AND ACTIVITIES

1.   Locate and read at least one article that describes an initiative that used a theoretical framework to design the intervention and one that did not use a theory. Draw the logic models for each. Review the conclusions for each initiative and discuss the authors' findings. What recommendations would you make to improve either or both initiatives?

2.   List the SMART attributes of objectives. Give two examples of SMART objectives.

3.   Describe how behavioral change and risk factors are related. Give an example of each and show how they help achieve a program goal.

4.   Develop a set of objectives to tackle the environmental factors that trigger a common health problem of your choice. What domains—individual, interpersonal, organizational, community, and public-policy—would you include, and what activities would you plan? What resources would you draw on?

5.   Draw a logic model that summarizes a program of your choice. Identify the outcomes you expect to achieve. Which theory would be useful for developing your initiative? Which stakeholders would you include, and how would you get them involved in your endeavor?

6.   Write a one-page summary of the social, economic, and political environments that would have an impact on the development of an initiative to address a public health problem in a community of your choice.

KEY TERMS

evidence-based initiatives	program activities
goals	SMART
logic models	stakeholders
mission	theory
objectives	Theory of Change

PLANNING FOR EVALUATION

LEARNING OBJECTIVES

- List the purposes of evaluation.
- Identify and describe the processes in managing an evaluation.
- Explain how evaluation standards and ethics underlie the evaluation process.
- Describe the role of stakeholders in evaluation planning.

The systematic collection of information about the activities and the outcomes of initiatives, which are an essential part of program evaluation, requires understanding the purposes and principles of evaluation as well as the appropriate management processes. This chapter describes how to plan an evaluation process.

When a group of program managers of public health initiatives were asked to define program evaluation they provided these two: "Evaluation means finding out important pieces of information that will help provide quality of service based on the needs of the target population." "Evaluation means a process for learning how a program was actually implemented and impacts of a program in the short and the long term."

Evaluation has these characteristics and more. Evaluation assesses the internal validity of an initiative and the extent to which an effect that is achieved is due to an intervention that was planned systematically. It is the cornerstone for improving public health initiatives because it provides information about the program through the conduct of culturally appropriate, carefully designed and executed research studies. The underlying assumption of public health interventions is that if an initiative is undertaken to address a problem through the conduct of a set of activities, the initiative will lead to a change in the participants or in the environment or in both. The initiative is assumed to cause the change, and therefore the intervention is effective and is understood to be worthy of the expenditure.

Evaluation is conducted for the purpose of making a judgment about a program's worth or value; it consists of a series of steps that must be matched with the needs of the project. The evaluation process is designed to answer a previously specified question by assessing the implementation of the program or policy and its outputs, outcomes, and impact. It provides feedback on the extent to which the initiative is achieving the organization's mission, goals, and objectives and makes recommendations for program improvements overall or for specific components of the program. In addition, evaluation studies attempt to determine whether the outcome was likely to have been caused by the initiative.

THE TIMING OF THE EVALUATION

Two considerations influence when an evaluation is carried out: first, whether the program is ready to be evaluated, and second, the stage of program development.

Readiness for Evaluation

The readiness for evaluation is assessed early in the process. This may take the form of a simple assessment of a detailed program plan and a Theory of Change; or it may be a more formal preassessment including evaluation of the data and the data-collection tools. In the Participatory Model of Evaluation, there is an excellent opportunity during the early discussions of the evaluation process and the contract to assess whether the program is ready for evaluation. The possibility of conducting the evaluation becomes clear once the program has been described and a Theory of Change and a logic model have been developed.

Stage of Development

The timing of the evaluation is also determined by the stage of development of the initiative, which in turn determines the evaluation design and implementation. A program in the early stages of development and within the first year or two requires a different evaluation approach, focus, and time line than a program that has been fully operational for ten years.

In the first year of a program, it is important to determine that the resources and program components are being implemented with fidelity and according to plan and the tools for measuring outcomes are put in place and are functioning appropriately. Outcomes are not assessed until the full implementation of the program or at specified intervals during the program in order to determine trends in a longitudinal study or a single outcome in a cross-sectional study.

THE PURPOSE OF EVALUATION

The purpose of an evaluation is generally to provide information for decision making or to provide information to improve evaluation practice.

- The evaluation may be undertaken in order to assess the extent to which the program is being implemented as planned or to determine whether the initiative is making or has made an impact on the beneficiaries.

- The evaluation may be undertaken in order to provide information for development of the initiative, to provide information for replication, or to determine its cost effectiveness compared with other programs.

- The evaluation may be undertaken in order to provide information about risk and protective factors or to assess alternative approaches for the prevention or treatment of health problems.

Although the primary purpose of an evaluation is to improve performance and to transform conditions, practice, structures, and systems, evaluations may serve other purposes:

- *Accountability* to the clients, community, funders, program management, and staff

- *Social justice* to ensure vulnerable populations receive appropriate and effective services

- *Program comparison* to determine best approaches

- *Evaluation research* to test a hypothesis

- *Program replication* at another site with another population

In the earliest stages of the development of the initiative, the purpose of the evaluation is to understand how the program or policy is being implemented or to assess whether the fully implemented initiative is likely to have the intended effect; such an assessment is known as a *formative evaluation*. Formative evaluation may be used in situations where the dynamics, the participants, and the issues change frequently and program activities must adjust to the changing environment. Formative evaluation provides early feedback and documentation to support a loop of assessment, planning, evaluation. Formative evaluation may be used to pretest educational materials and initiative components. It answers the following questions:

- Do the program components work effectively?

- What are the factors that influence program implementation favorably and unfavorably?

- Is the program culturally appropriate?

When the purpose of the evaluation is to determine whether the program or policy is being implemented appropriately or the extent to which the program is being implemented, it is known as a *process evaluation*. It focuses on reviewing documentation of implementation such as logs, meeting notes, registration documents. It may review data-collection processes and outputs. It may also involve interviewing participants or project personnel. Improving the program or work in progress is the purpose of process evaluation. Major questions during this phase include:

- Is the program/intervention being implemented according to the plan that was laid out before the program started?

- What type, quantity, and quality of services are being provided?

- What are staffing and training levels?

- How many meetings and trainings are held and for whom?

- Who is participating and how?

If the purpose of the evaluation is to determine the effect of the program or policy, then it is known as an *outcome evaluation*. An outcome evaluation is performed at the end of the intervention or after a predetermined time during program implementation. The appropriate time for an outcome evaluation is determined by the time line associated with the program objectives, by the completion of the program, or, in the case of a policy initiative, after the policy has been in place for an extended period. Outcome evaluations answer questions such as these:

- Did the program or policy make a difference and produce a change in those affected directly by it?

- What results were produced by the initiative over time?

- What changes in knowledge, attitudes, beliefs, or behavior were produced in those who participated?

- What changes occurred in the environment as a result of the initiative?

- What trends occurred in the incidence of the public health problem over time?

If the purpose of the evaluation is to determine whether initiatives have contributed to a population-level effect, it is known as an *impact evaluation*. The terms *outcome* and *impact* are often used interchangeably within different sectors of public health. In this book, *outcome* is used for short-, medium-, and long-term changes that occur during the first few years of program or policy implementation. *Impact* is used for long-term changes in quality of life that occur at the local, state, and national levels, that are detected using surveillance methods, and that occur in the population at large from a plethora of activities that occur over time in multiple sectors. An impact evaluation answers this question: Did all the efforts of the combined initiatives influence rates of disease, disability, or mortality, or the quality of life of the residents?

The purpose of an evaluation also may be *cost-benefit* or *cost-effectiveness analyses*, which allow evaluators to determine whether the cost associated with the program is worth the investment. These analyses answer this question: What were the benefits of the program relative to the expenditures?

ESTABLISHING THE CONTRACT FOR EVALUATION

The evaluation contract is negotiated by the initiator—the funding agency, the board of directors, the executive director, or other person designated by the agency. If the organization has an internal evaluator, that person may be given the responsibility to conduct the evaluation. In most cases, however, an external evaluator is identified through local or national searches or through personal contacts.

The lead evaluator has primary responsibility for the evaluation and negotiates the terms based on previous experience, knowledge, skills, and orientation. The contract, which may be in the form of a letter or a formal legal document, contains the following:

- Name of the evaluator (as contractor) and the name of the contracting agent

- Statement of the purpose of the evaluation

- Statements about access to management and staff, initiative beneficiaries, resources, and logistics for the time period during which the evaluation will be carried out

- Specific expectations for reports and other documentation of the evaluation

- Amount budgeted for the evaluation

- Time line for the evaluation

- Dated signatures of all parties to the contract

THE EVALUATION TEAM

Following the execution of the contract, the lead evaluator, working with the contracting organization, identifies members of the evaluation team. The team should include stakeholders with the expertise to develop and implement the evaluation plan, although roles may shift during the evaluation process and training may be required for community members.

The evaluation team must have evaluation expertise in multiple areas and the knowledge and skills required for completing the task. The size of the team is often determined by the budget. If necessary, ad hoc teams may be formed to carry out specific tasks related to the evaluation. A commitment to training stakeholders and to providing the necessary skills during the process is likely to lead people to participate (Travers et al., 2008). Such a commitment ensures equity across the team and buy-in from the start and is likely to lead to the organization's using the findings (Patton, 2008). People on the evaluation team should include those with skills in

- working across disciplines

- cross-cultural communication

- critical thinking and evaluation

- research methodology

- data collection

- data management, analysis, and interpretation

- technical writing and reporting

As part of effective evaluation practice, the lead evaluator should ask who is not at the table, which voices will not be heard, and why. The team should make every effort to include those voices in the process.

The contributions of the stakeholders include providing an understanding of the program, providing input into the development of the evaluation plan, providing support to the implementation of the plan through data collection and analysis, and providing input into the interpretation of the results and writing the final report.

The evaluation-team leader has ultimate responsibility for ensuring the integrity of the evaluation process and that it is carried out with the highest ethical standards and is completed within the agreed-on time frame. The evaluator should "ensure that the evaluation team collectively possesses the evaluation abilities, skills, and experience appropriate to the evaluation" (American Evaluation Association, 2008, p. 233).

Once the team is assembled, the first step is to orient everyone to the team's approach to the evaluation. It is particularly important to orient the community members and newcomers to the art and science of evaluation. Encouraging evaluative thinking as part of the community's or the organization's culture increases the likelihood that data collection for evaluation purposes is incorporated systematically into initiatives (Patton, 2008).

The team must work through multiple steps in the process to complete the terms of the contract and provide the expected products within the specified time. It must define a plan of action with multiple components and steps that describe the activities that the team will undertake to complete the evaluation. Completing the evaluation requires the development of a well-functioning and effective team.

CREATING AND MAINTAINING EFFECTIVE PARTNERSHIPS

Effective partnership development is as critical for program evaluation as it is for the outside community and its institutions. Panet-Raymond (1992) suggests that partnerships are successful when they have

- established power and legitimacy (and strive for an equitable relationship)

- well-defined missions, a clear sense of purpose, and common goals

- respect for each other, and clear expectations of the partnership

- commitment to the partnership approach

- open-mindedness, patience, respect, and sensitivity

In addition, partners benefit from having written agreements clarifying objectives, responsibilities, methods, and approaches for the partnership and its work (Panet-Raymond, 1992).

Establishing and maintaining healthy partnerships can be both difficult and time consuming, yet the partnership is critical for participatory evaluation and must be nurtured (Fitzpatrick et al., 2004). Suggestions for nurturing the partnership include the following:

- Prepare evaluation sponsors and other stakeholders by framing evaluation in an understandable way.

- Encourage and support stakeholder participation and teamwork.

- Plan sufficient time for the evaluation process.

- Encourage and support active participation of stakeholders.

Stakeholder support and participation is enhanced through providing multiple opportunities for input throughout the evaluation process. Such input occurs when stakeholders have wide and varied experiences, knowledge, and skills, and when they have been provided with appropriate and timely training. Constructive critique and negotiation are also important strategies (Fitzpatrick et al., 2004).

In successful groups, members rely on each other and involve each other in planning and decision making. Achieving a common goal also requires that the group members possess task-related and positive socioemotional behaviors (Belcher, 1994). Task-related behaviors include providing opinions, evaluations, suggestions, and information or asking for suggestions, direction, opinions, or analysis. Positive socioemotional behaviors are showing solidarity, helping, showing satisfaction, laughing, and joking. In contrast, negative socioemotional behaviors are disagreeing, withholding help, showing tension, showing antagonism, defending or asserting oneself while deflating another's status (Belcher, 1994).

Effective communication is critical for maintaining effective group dynamics. Such communication includes listening carefully and attentively to what other people are saying. It may mean paraphrasing to ensure understanding of what is being said. It also includes being attentive to body language and how it affects the interaction. When we look at the person we are talking to, we indicate that we are listening. Looking away or walking away indicates that we are not listening. The approaches that are selected for communication are important and must take into consideration culture, reading levels, and language preferences.

Developing cultural competence to work with groups and with communities is a life-long process that requires examining one's own biases. It requires avoiding the use of stereotypes and recognizing that within cultures there are also individuals who may embody some but not all aspects of the culture that is being defined. Often we consider Hispanic culture to be monolithic and ignore the fact that within the group there are multiple subgroups. Likewise we may assume that all blacks are the same; however blacks may come from a variety of continents and countries with their own cultures. Cross-cultural communication and developing cultural competence require that we also understand that within each cultural group there are social networks that support and protect its people.

Both the community partners and the evaluators face challenges in the community-engagement process and in working in teams, and yet there are opportunities to learn through it all. I teach an award-winning evaluation class that requires students to conduct an evaluation in a local community-based organization or public health agency. The students work with coaches from the community organizations to answer one or two evaluation questions. Students are asked to write down their reflections of their involvement in the project. One of my students said of the experience, "I have never been put into a situation like the community evaluation project that required me to use critical thinking and problem solving skills for a variety of situations—whether it was communication problems we were having or problems when developing our suggested tool for our organization to use."

The community partners may face challenges of their own. Another student in her reflections made the following observation: "I was expecting these organizations and coaches to be very welcoming and excited about our work for their project. But instead I realize that maybe some organizations are a little fearful of what these evaluations will expose about how the organization is functioning. I try to put myself in their shoes, and think how would I react if I learned I wasn't doing what I claimed or what I was supposed to be doing, and, all along, I thought I was doing a great job. That would be very difficult."

Dealing with these challenges is part of the process of developing an evaluation team, and using the participatory process of evaluation allows the team to take the time to help stakeholders understand the merits of conducting an evaluation. It also allows time for issues to be resolved. The challenges of engaging stakeholders in the evaluation process are offset by the gains that are achieved that make the team stronger and ensure a useful product.

EVALUATION STANDARDS

The public health community adopted a set of evaluation standards (Milstein et al., 2000) put forward by the Joint Commission on Standards for Educational Evaluation (Joint Committee on Standards for Educational Evaluation, Sanders, & American

Association of School Administrators, 1994; Patton, 2008) that inform the practice of public health today. The broad concepts of the standards of evaluation practice are utility, feasibility, propriety, and accuracy.

Utility: The utility standard requires that the information provided by the evaluation be useful to the stakeholders and those who will use the results. It addresses the amount and type of information that is collected, the interpretation of evaluation findings, as well as when and how the final report is produced. It encourages evaluation to be planned, conducted, and reported in ways that increase the likelihood of stakeholders' using the evaluation findings.

Feasibility: The feasibility standard requires that the evaluation process be practical and nondisruptive, that it acknowledge the political nature of the evaluation, and that resources that are available for conducting the evaluation be used carefully to produce results. It specifies that evaluations should be efficient and produce information that justifies the expense.

Propriety: The propriety standard requires that the evaluation be ethical and be conducted with regard for the rights of those involved and affected. It requires that the evaluation be complete and fair in its process and reporting. It also requires that the evaluation demonstrate respect for human dignity and avoid conflicts of interest; it cites the Tuskegee syphilis study as a reminder of the evaluators' responsibilities.

Accuracy: The accuracy standard requires that the evaluation use accurate and systematic processes for conducting qualitative and quantitative research and that it produce technically accurate conclusions that are defensible and justifiable.

MANAGING THE EVALUATION PROCESS

An important consideration for evaluators is how an evaluation plan will be implemented and how the research will be managed. Evaluation projects are organized into four major phases. The first one is to recruit an evaluation team; the second is to review and confirm the terms of the contract and to make decisions regarding supervision and finances; the third is to develop an evaluation research plan; and the fourth is to develop a budget for the evaluation.

Recruiting and Developing Team Members

The first task of the lead evaluator is to recruit and assemble a team of people who will conduct the evaluation. The evaluation focus and the methods and funding determine team membership and the expertise required of team members. It is important to develop a multidisciplinary team for cross-discipline initiative evaluations that involve multiple domains. An evaluation that requires conducting a cost analysis may require different skills than one that requires the assessment of behavioral outcomes. The team must assess the needs of each evaluation carefully and throughout the process. If during the evaluation process new skills are needed, the evaluator must consider increasing the membership, either permanently or by using consultants. This decision will usually have funding implications that must be weighed carefully also. As teams change, it is also important to address issues that influence and change the dynamics of the group and decision making; ensuring equitable participation of team members is essential.

Once the team is recruited and assembled, the next step is to identify tasks for team members. Decisions regarding training and building skills to complete evaluation tasks must be made at this time. Training may be formal or informal depending on the needs of the project.

Deciding on Contract Terms, Supervision, and Finances

The Contract   Because the evaluation contract provides only a brief overview of the evaluation and its product, the evaluation team needs to discuss and negotiate the details and the expectations with the clients and other stakeholders. The team has many responsibilities during these sessions:

- Discuss and decide on the overarching and specific evaluation research question(s). This discussion may cover previous evaluations of the program. An assessment of findings may provide insights and help identify questions that could be included in a new evaluation.

- Discuss data-collection options and access to research participants.

- Understand the climate for conducting the evaluation. Politically charged climates may make evaluation challenging. The team needs to understand the dynamics between the client and other local, state, and national stakeholders. These may include relationships with the board, funders, and the competition.

- Review the budget and determine the scope and scale of the evaluation. It is important to spend time developing a well-thought-out budget for the evaluation that will be adhered to closely. Evaluations are generally not well funded, and going back to the client for more money is usually not an option for the evaluation team, unless the scope of work changes significantly at the request of the client. If it is possible, the team should build in a review process to allow that flexibility and also should build in agreements with regard to moving expenditures within the budget—for example, from supplies to travel. If such changes need to be made, it is important to contact the funder. Generally, changes of 10 percent are easily allowed.

- Identify roles and responsibilities for members of the evaluation team, staff, and key stakeholders. Discuss the principles of the participatory approach to conducting the evaluation and get buy-in.

- Identify the logistics for the evaluation (support staff, office supplies, transportation, meeting space, data resources). Discuss how data bases, reports, and publications will be made accessible to the evaluation team. This discussion may cover time frames and personnel. Staff is often busy and find it difficult to accommodate the requests of evaluators, so allow plenty of time for requests to be honored.

- Discuss ownership of the evaluation data. Unlike data from traditional research projects, evaluation data often belong to the client. It is important to clarify data ownership early in the process to avoid any misunderstanding later. This discussion should also cover publication of the findings. Permission may need to be obtained to report at conferences and in other ways publish the findings.

- Discuss the expectations during the period of the evaluation for interim and final reports and check-ins, including formats and mechanisms for reporting.

Supervision   Managing an evaluation project can be time consuming and requires different although complementary skills. It entails supervising staff and volunteers at each stage of the process as well as the day-to-day coordination of the team's efforts. It may include identifying and securing resources and ensuring that deadlines are met and deliverables are developed. It may also require setting up meetings, following up on project commitments, and writing reports. In most evaluations, the management functions are carried out by the evaluator or a member of the team, but when the project is large, such as a statewide evaluation, it may be necessary to hire a project manager whose sole responsibility is coordination. When hiring a project manager, the skills of the individual are matched with the requirements of the specific evaluation.

Finances   During this period the team must also consider how the finances will be handled. The team leader will usually have the final responsibility for ensuring funds are spent appropriately, but mechanisms should be designed to monitor and track spending. The level of monitoring and tracking will depend on the size, duration, and complexity of the project. The more complex the evaluation is, the more likely it is that an accountant needs to be involved.

Developing the Evaluation Research Plan

After the contract is signed by all parties, convene the evaluation team and develop a detailed evaluation research plan. This plan will contain a number of components:

- Project design

- Data collection and management

- Dissemination of findings

Project Design   Undertaking the evaluation research project entails selecting the most appropriate design for answering the evaluation research question. The design is determined by the stage of the program to be evaluated, the evaluation question that is to be answered, the budget, the expertise of the team, and the time line.

The team develops a project action plan that encapsulates the project design. For the evaluation as a whole and for each major component, the action plan outlines the activities and the time frame for completing them. As the project continues. the team may need different action plans that will fall within the scope of the project action plan. An action plan provides a graphic representation of the time line and required tasks and may also designate responsible persons. It differs from a logic model in that a logic model is a graphic representation of the initiative's Theory of Change; the logic model outlines the assumed links among the health problem, the activities used to resolve it, and the expected outcomes of the intervention. Examples of a basic action plan and of a plan for team recruitment and development are provided in Tables 4.1 and 4.2. Consider also using project-management software, which facilitates the development and management of the plans.

TABLE 4.1. **A Basic Action Plan**

Major Project Activities	1st Quarter	2nd Quarter	3rd Quarter	4th Quarter
1. Team recruitment and development	x			
2. Make contract, supervision, and financial decisions	x			
3. Project design	x	x		
4. Data collection and management			x	
5. Dissemination of findings				x

TABLE 4.2. **An Action Plan for Team Recruitment and Development**

Team Recruitment and Development	1st Quarter			Responsible Person(s)
	Month 1	Month 2	Month 3	
• Identify potential team members	x			
• Invite stakeholders to be on the team	x	x		
• Conduct orientation for team members			x	

Data Collection and Management Based on the design selected and the type of questions to be answered, the most appropriate data-collection methods are identified. In an optimal evaluation:

▓ The best data-collection methods are used.

▓ The data that are collected are both valid and reliable.

▓ The analysis of the data is appropriate and accurate.

Selecting the best approach to data collection and the best data requires that researchers be oriented toward the specifics of the project; hence, training must be built into the time line and the budget. Divisions of the National Institutes of Health, the Centers for Disease Control and Prevention, and foundations now fund Community-Based Participatory Research intervention projects that require the involvement of multiple partners, many of whom have no experience with research. Members of the community who form part of the team and others who want to participate in the evaluation may need extensive training to develop their skills in research and data collection and in data analysis.

In addition, the data-collection approach selected must be credible and provide valid and reliable data. The evaluation team assesses the options and decides on the most appropriate methods. It develops or assembles appropriate data-collection instruments and decides on the needs for analysis, which may include personnel and logistics. Once the evaluation project is complete a final step is evaluating the evaluation itself to understand the strengths and weaknesses of the design, data collection, and the evaluation process overall. This evaluation assesses the validity of the conclusions and their relevance to stakeholders.

Dissemination of Findings As the evaluation team plans the evaluation, it must also discuss important aspects of the dissemination of the results, including:

▓ The stakeholders' expectations of how the results will be used

▓ The timing of evaluation reports that may be provided periodically during the evaluation process or at the end as a final report

▓ The audience characteristics that will influence the presentation formats and style

Budgeting for the Evaluation

Using the budget approved in the contract process, the team develops a working budget that is based on the specifics of the evaluation plan. Table 4.3 is a sample budget. It includes costs for personnel, equipment and supplies, printing, and participants. The data-collection approach may have additional costs associated with it. A budget justification explains each budget line. For example, it specifies the number of staff, the level of staff, and the salary and benefits. In the table, the project coordinator earns $60,000 per year with fringe benefits at 23 percent and works on the evaluation 10 percent of the time.

TABLE 4.3. **Sample Budget**

Budget Item	YR 1$	YR 2$	YR 3	YR 4	YR 5
Staff Salaries and Benefits Project coordinator (1) 10% @ $60,000 + 23% Interviewers (2) 25% @ $50,000 + 23% Data analyst (1) 50% @ $50,000 + 23%	119,925	125,921			
Consultant Fees (if required) 10 days @ $200 per day	2,000	2,100			
Travel (project team and study participants) Out of state $2,000 In state $5,000	7,000	7,000			
Equipment and Supplies Computer $1,300 Software $1,500 General office supplies $1,000	3,800	1,000			
Communication Internet Telephone	1,800	2,000			
Participants Stipends $500 Transcriptions 15 @ $300 per interview	5,000	5,000			
Printing Surveys 200 @ $.50 per copy	100	100			
Photocopying	100	100			
Subtotal	139,725	143,221			
Indirect costs (depending on funder) @ 25%	34,931	35,805			
TOTAL	$174,656	$179,026			

The budget will reflect the cost of the project director with a possible increase in succeeding years. The cost of equipment and supplies in this example decreases in succeeding years because computer and software expenses are necessary in the first year only.

FACTORS THAT INFLUENCE THE EVALUATION PROCESS

A well-designed and implemented program or policy evaluation depends on a variety of factors that the evaluation team may have more or less control over. It is important that the evaluation team consider the possible limitations in order to provide the most cost-sensitive and useful evaluation.

Factors That Cannot Be Controlled

Factors that may influence an evaluation but that the evaluators have limited or no control over include:

▦ *The level of funding and of the resources allocated for the evaluation*. The higher the funding and the more resources available for the evaluation the more comprehensive the evaluation will be.

▦ *Personnel support*. An adequate level of support is important to ensure access to resources, to the study population, to data, and to logistics that support the evaluation.

▦ *The time line*. One that limits the type of data or the quantity of data that can be collected will limit the evaluation.

▦ *Access to the study population and to program data*. The degree of access may influence a number of parameters of the evaluation. It may affect the amount and the quality of the data that are collected; low amounts and poor quality of data introduce bias and affect the validity of the study. A sociopolitical environment with little or no support for the evaluation makes the process difficult and results in difficulty in collecting the information, limited access to resources, and difficulty in sharing and utilizing evaluation findings. The sociopolitical environment is influenced by who requested the evaluation and who has a vested interest in the results.

Factors That Can Be Controlled

There are also factors that the evaluator has control over and must take into consideration during the planning process. These factors may include the level and type of expertise on the evaluation team and the management of the evaluation process.

Level and Type of Expertise on the Evaluation Team   The level and type of expertise on the evaluation team will influence the type of evaluation that is conducted and access to the study population. It is important to ensure that members of the team have knowledge and skills to contribute to some part of the process, while recognizing that not all members will contribute to all parts of the evaluation. For example, a stakeholder may be influential in the community but may know nothing about the evaluation process. Nevertheless, he or she may be able to contribute significantly to developing the research tools and to providing input to ensure the tools and approaches are sensitive to the study population. That member may also be instrumental in another stage of the process, recruiting members of the community to complete the surveys and participate in the focus groups or in photography and digital storytelling. Without that member's contributions, the evaluation may take longer than planned and may even not collect valid and reliable data.

The evaluation team also requires skills in evaluation, which will depend on the nature of the project to be evaluated. If, for example, the evaluation calls for a cost-benefit analysis in addition to the usual outcome evaluation, it is important that the team recruit a member who has skills in conducting such an analysis or that the team be willing to pay a consultant for that expertise.

Whether the required knowledge and skills are available on the evaluation team will determine its success. Recruiting the right people and providing the requisite training are crucial.

Management of the Evaluation Process   Apart from having the appropriate expertise on the evaluation team, the team must also be managed appropriately to complete the project and fulfill the requirements of the contract. For example, if the agreement is to provide a mid-year interim report to coincide with a mid-year review of the project by the board of directors, the evaluation team has the responsibility for meeting that deadline. To do so, the team has to complete all the tasks of data collection and data analysis and write a report that is appropriate given the status of the project.

INVOLVING STAKEHOLDERS

All those who have an interest in the program and the evaluation are the stakeholders and the audience for the evaluation. They are involved in both the process and the management of the evaluation. As mentioned above, extensive stakeholder involvement increases the level of oversight for the evaluation project, improves its credibility, and increases the likelihood that the evaluation results will be used. As in previous components of conducting the evaluation, stakeholders play a critical part in designing the evaluation. They are important contributors to

- framing and selecting the appropriate evaluation questions

- identifying the concepts that are critical to measure

- developing and executing the evaluation plan

In this participatory evaluation and empowerment, model all members of the evaluation team advance their knowledge and skills during critical thinking and decision-making processes that go on throughout. It is important for the team to

- choose the most important and appropriate evaluation questions for making decisions and improving effectiveness

- balance the need to assess implementation and process with the need to assess effectiveness and outcomes

- select the most appropriate measures, approaches, and tools, taking into consideration the expertise of the group, time frames, and the budget

SUMMARY

- Creating effective partnerships for evaluation requires effective cross-cultural communication; participation and teamwork; shared goals; and open-mindedness, patience, and sensitivity.

- Initiatives go through stages of development that determine the type of evaluation and the design of the evaluation. Process and outcome are types of evaluation that occur at different stages.

- The evaluation process includes specifying the initiative, the inputs, the outputs, and the outcomes that define the success of the intervention and specifying the methodology for collecting the information (data), for analyzing the data, and for disseminating the results so they are useful to the stakeholders.

- The type of evaluation is determined by the stage of development of the program. In the early stages of development and within the first year or two, a formative or process evaluation is required. After the program is fully implemented and stable, an outcome evaluation is generally undertaken. An outcome evaluation may be complemented by a process evaluation.

- Establishing and maintaining healthy partnerships can be both difficult and time consuming, yet partnerships are critical for participatory evaluation and must be nurtured.

- The evaluation standards put forward by the Joint Commission on Standards for Educational Evaluation are utility, feasibility, propriety, and accuracy.

DISCUSSION QUESTIONS AND ACTIVITIES

1. Imagine you are the executive director of a large, not-for-profit organization that has multiple initiatives and has just received new funding for up to five years to address a single public health problem. You would like an evaluation plan developed for your organization. You do not have the expertise to carry out an evaluation yourself, but you know what needs to be done. What would be the advantages and disadvantages of hiring an external evaluator versus asking the person in your organization who is in charge of the data center to conduct the evaluation of the new initiatives?

2. Discuss the implications of using the standards of evaluation practice in developing an evaluation plan for a program of your choice offered by a community-based, youth-serving, minority organization with limited funding.

3. Imagine you have been invited to join a team to conduct an evaluation of a local advocacy organization in a rural part of the state. What knowledge and skills would you consider important for effective team process?

KEY TERMS

accuracy

contract

cost-benefit or cost-effectiveness analysis

cross-cultural communication

evaluation standards

feasibility

formative evaluation

hypothesis

impact evaluation

inputs

outcome evaluation

outcomes

outputs

process evaluation

propriety

utility

CHAPTER

5

DESIGNING THE EVALUATION

DESCRIBING THE PROGRAM

LEARNING OBJECTIVES

- Explain why it is necessary to have a systematic process for describing a program.

- Describe the components involved in describing a program.

- Explain the importance of a logic model in program evaluation.

The participatory model described in this book identifies a four-step approach for ensuring a systematic evaluation (Figure 5.1):

1. Design the evaluation.

2. Collect the data.

3. Analyze and interpret the data.

4. Report the findings.

In order to perform the first step, designing the evaluation, it is important that the program be well described and understood by each member of the evaluation team. This chapter explains how to describe the public health initiative; the next chapter explains the other tasks in designing an evaluation: how to identify the research question and specify the evaluation research design.

Describing the initiative, its development, and its context allows stakeholders and the evaluation team to reach a common understanding so that appropriate research questions can be asked and answered. The stakeholders are critical in this process as they are likely to know the most about their programs. This process is time consuming and requires patience. It is important to get multiple perspectives, as each stakeholder may view the program from a different standpoint. If the initiative has changed since the planning documents were written, the chances are the initiative being evaluated is significantly different.

The importance of carefully describing a program to be evaluated is often not fully appreciated by new and seasoned evaluators alike. An initiative needs to be described for three reasons. First, describing the program provides evaluators with an understanding of

FIGURE 5.1. *The Participatory Framework for Evaluation: Design the Evaluation*

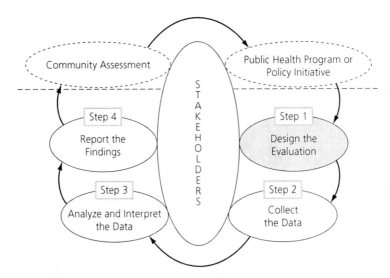

the program's ability to produce the changes that are outlined in the goals and objectives (Centers for Disease Control and Prevention, 1999). Second, clear descriptions of programs are required for meeting the program evaluation standards of utility and accuracy (Joint Committee on Standards for Educational Evaluation et al., 1994). Third, describing the initiative supports the development of recommendations at the end of the process.

During this stage of designing the program, the program is described in several ways: by describing the context of the initiative; the justifications for the initiative; the initiative's goals, objectives, and activities; and the initiative's Theory of Change and logic model.

THE CONTEXT

The first component in understanding the organization's context is to understand its mission as contained in the mission statement. The mission statement defines in clear terms what the organization sets out to do.

The second component to understanding the organization's context is to understand the social, political, and economic climate in which it operates. This climate defines what the organization can and cannot do and the level of support it has for the initiatives it wants to offer. For example, in a low-income neighborhood with poor social and economic conditions, it may not be expedient to offer programs that may be politically unpopular. The economic context and therefore current and past funding levels may shed light on the initiative's local and national support and its long-term sustainability. Other aspects of the organization's social, political, and economic climate include its budget, assets, and the resources available to it and to the community at large for addressing the problem.

The third component to understanding the organization's context is to understand its structure. Generally a nonprofit organization has a board of directors that oversees its programming and provides recommendations for the organization's direction. Public agencies might have advisory bodies that provide recommendations. Other parts of an organization's structure are the staffing arrangements and the responsibilities of critical staff like the executive director and other directors and senior managers.

EXAMPLE

MISSION
STATEMENT

"To eliminate social and economic barriers to good health through policy change and evidenced-based initiatives by collaboration among communities and organizations."

Understanding staffing arrangements includes understanding work responsibilities and time and effort implementing the activities of the initiative.

In order to understand an organization's structure, the evaluation team can create an organizational chart (Figure 5.2 is an example) showing lines of authority. The figure presents the structure of a nonprofit organization overseen by a board of directors; the organization, with thirty-five staff members, has five funded initiatives. The executive director supervises four directors, one each for policy initiatives, finance, programs, and public relations. The office of the director of finance has an accounts manager, and the program coordinator reports directly to the director of programs. The program and volunteer staff are supervised by the program coordinator.

The fourth component to understanding the organization's context is to understand the initiative's structure and its relationship to the organization. So, for example, if the initiative that is being evaluated is one of three programs, then it is important to understand how they relate to each other, specifically with regard to staff-time distributions, supervision, and funding.

In addition, the team of evaluators studies

- the characteristics of the initiative that make it appropriate for addressing the problem

- the features of the initiative that address the particular needs of the population as defined by age, gender, ethnicity, and culture

FIGURE 5.2.   *Organizational Chart*

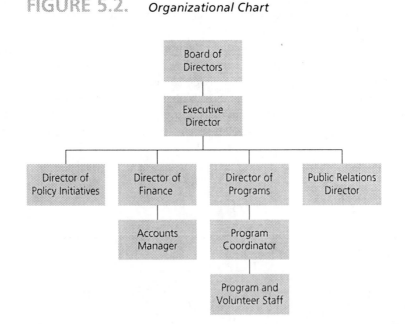

▧ the training and preparation of the program staff and their capacity to undertake the initiative

Additional questions, including the following, may help evaluators make an informed decision about the initiative's merits:

▧ How does the initiative reflect and build on the assets, strengths, and attributes of the community?

▧ To what extent is this intervention compatible with other programs within the organization?

▧ To what extent does the intervention complement or build on existing programs?

▧ To what extent does this initiative contribute to the community's overall public health goal?

In conducting an evaluation of an initiative, it is important to review ethical issues and issues of social justice. Evaluators should

▧ assess whether the program is developmentally and culturally appropriate for the intended population

▧ assess whether the initiative is being delivered in a fair, equitable, and respectful manner

▧ determine whether members of the intended population are involved in program planning and development

▧ determine whether members of the intended population are participating in the initiative

▧ assess whether populations who could benefit from the initiative are being left out

The fifth component to understanding the organization's context is to understand how data are collected and how they are utilized to draw conclusions. Evaluators need to know the type of data, the quality and quantity of data, and the level of sophistication of the data-management systems. The level of sophistication may range from simple—a paper system with scratch pads for case histories—to sophisticated, in which all data are entered in a data base by each member of staff. The more advanced the system is, the more technically complex monitoring the organization can undertake.

JUSTIFICATIONS FOR THE INITIATIVE

In justifying the initiative's development, the extent to which the public health problem affects sectors of the population and the factors that contribute to its existence at the individual, community, organizational, and policy level are assessed. During this phase in describing the program, the administrators and staff are asked about the motivations for the program. These justifications can sometimes be found in the organization's reports of community assessments or other documents. The results of the community assessments may be published in agency, local, state, or national reports and may have been used for program or policy development.

In addition to reviewing existing data and reports, the team conducts a review of epidemiological studies published in the scientific literature to determine the incidence, prevalence, morbidity, disability, and mortality rates associated with the problem in the nation, in the state, and in the community of interest. Such a review provides a means to compare the program being evaluated with others that are similar. The literature review also provides information on the social, cultural, and environmental conditions associated with the public health problem. It describes in narrative form the nature of the problem, those who are affected by it, and why, how, and when they were affected, and it provides guidance for assessing the risk and protective factors associated with the problem at the individual, interpersonal, and environmental levels and also the social determinants of health that influence the problem. The review of the scientific literature is part of the introduction in the evaluation report described in Chapter Eleven.

THE INITIATIVE'S GOALS, OBJECTIVES, AND ACTIVITIES

In addition to describing the justifications for the program, the evaluation team describes the expected effects of the intervention. These are stated as the initiatives' goal and objectives, as described in Chapter Three.

If there are no clearly defined objectives for the initiative, the evaluators work with stakeholders to define expected outcomes for the program and to formulate objectives that can be used for evaluation. The baseline for the objectives may be obtained from the description of similar initiatives in the literature or in reported research. This search may also yield targets for the intervention. Healthy People 2010 (U.S. Department of Health and Human Services, 2000) provides national targets, while the Millennium Development Goals 2015 (United Nations, 2008) provides international targets that may also be adopted. Without objectives, evaluators are in the dark regarding the targets for evaluation.

THE INITIATIVE'S THEORY OF CHANGE AND LOGIC MODEL

The evaluation team describes the initiative in terms of the perceived Theory of Change and the logic model (see Chapter Three). The Theory of Change is discussed with the stakeholders to clarify understanding and allow for further input. It is important to evaluators for several reasons:

▪ It provides a shared understanding of the program.

▪ It provides a tool for discussion among a diverse group of stakeholders.

▪ It clarifies the benchmarks and intended effects of the program.

- It documents program activities and program resources.

- It provides opportunities to discuss strengths and weaknesses of program components.

The final step in describing the program is developing the program's logic model, which depicts its resources, activities, outputs, and outcomes in a graphic way. (Figure 5.3 is an example.) The logic model provides the team with a shared understanding of the program components and forms the foundation for the development of the evaluation process. The logic model clearly articulates the program's Theory of Change, which may be tested in the evaluation. The logic model provides a framework from which to identify evaluation questions. Logic models can be developed to support different aspects of the program and to suit different purposes (Centers for Disease Control and Prevention, 1999). For example, if the initiative has multiple activities, then each set of activities can form the basis for an additional logic model depicting its resources, outputs, and short-, medium-, and long-term outcomes.

During the developmental phases of a program or when new components are added to an initiative, the logic model may change. It is important to revisit and update the initiative's logic model periodically so that it provides an accurate representation of the initiative being evaluated. In the complex world of public health, there may be a need to update the components represented in the logic model as the program matures and changes.

FIGURE 5.3.   *Logic Model for a Program to Train Older Adults as Companions*

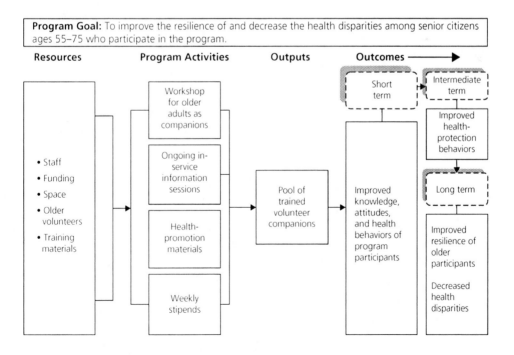

Program Goal: To improve the resilience of and decrease the health disparities among senior citizens ages 55–75 who participate in the program.

SUMMARY

▪ Describing the initiative provides an understanding of the social, cultural, economic, political, and structural context of the organization. It supports the development of recommendations at the end of the process. Knowing a program's strengths and weaknesses allows the team to develop a feasible and useful evaluation.

▪ A thorough understanding of the program is achieved only from the multiple perspectives of the program's administrators, funders, staff, and advocates, as well as its current and past participants.

▪ A logic model provides a tool for stakeholders so that they can have a shared understanding of the initiative, can clarify benchmarks, and can identify strengths and weaknesses.

DISCUSSION QUESTIONS AND ACTIVITIES

1. Describe a public health initiative's organizational, sociocultural, political, and economic contexts. What questions might stakeholders have that would guide an evaluation?

2. Contact a local community-based organization that focuses on policy or the environment. Draw a logic model that provides a graphic representation of the Theory of Change for one of the organization's initiatives and describe what you learn about the initiative from doing so.

KEY TERMS

activities   objectives
goals   Theory of Change

6

DESIGNING THE EVALUATION

LEARNING OBJECTIVES

▪ Describe how to choose a process or outcome evaluation question.

▪ Describe evaluation research designs.

▪ List and describe the threats to internal and external validity.

In addition to describing the program, stakeholders identify the evaluation questions in the first step of the participatory model (designing the evaluation). Evaluation questions guide the evaluation team in conducting the research to fulfill the primary purpose of an evaluation: to gain insight into the initiative and how it is implemented or to assess its effects. The evaluation question drives the research design and the data-collection methods. Without an evaluation question, there really is no evaluation!

Evaluation questions must

- be clear and specify what is being assessed

- be linked directly to the program or policy being implemented

- be linked to indicators that allow for direct or indirect measurement

- incorporate the needs and expectations of stakeholders

The logic model may be used as the starting point for identifying evaluation questions, as illustrated in Figure 6.1. The assembled evaluation team and other stakeholders

FIGURE 6.1. *Logic-Model Framework for Identifying Evaluation Questions*

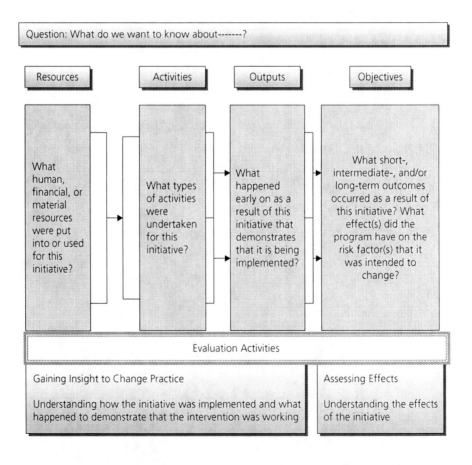

make their way across the logic model from left to right. At each stage the question asked is, What do we want to know? For example, in the resources box the question might be, What resources were provided for the initiative or a part of the initiative? In the outputs box, the questions might be, How satisfied are our clients? or How many and which clients did we serve?

However, stakeholders may want to assess the effects of the program on the participants. They may have questions such as, What changes occurred in the participants? or, Were participants in the initiative more successful than those who did not participate? or, What effect did the enactment of the policy have on underage drinking?

BASES FOR SELECTING THE EVALUATION QUESTIONS

The evaluation research questions are based on

- the concerns and priorities of the stakeholders

- the components of the logic model

- the initiative's previously developed outcome and activity objectives

- the expertise of the evaluation team

The Concerns and Priorities of the Stakeholders

Stakeholders' expectations of the program may be different from the stated objectives. In a recent evaluation the following questions were identified by a stakeholder:

1. Are customers purchasing fruits and vegetables more frequently since the intervention has taken place? At the store? In total?

2. Which food items are selling the most?

3. Has the store profited from the sales of fresh produce?

These questions led to considering a number of factors about the evaluation, the stage of the initiative, the evaluation design, and the data-collection methodology.

Components of the Logic Model

The components of the logic model may help frame evaluation questions. The logic model is an excellent tool for thinking through the most appropriate elements to measure. Each box in the logic model provides opportunities for evaluation. Evaluation questions related to inputs allow the evaluation team to assess what resources went into the program as well as what resources were expended as a result of the program. This is valuable information in the conduct of a cost-benefit analysis or for purposes of accounting or replication.

Outputs are also useful to determine. They provide first indications that the program is working. If, as in Figure 6.2, the goal of the program is to reduce the incidence of obesity among children, one of the outcome objectives would be to increase access to fresh fruits and vegetables; the activity objective would then be to organize farmers'

FIGURE 6.2. *Relationship Between Outcome and Activity Objectives and Outputs*

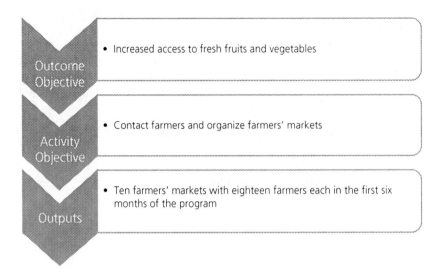

markets. The Theory of Action for the initiative suggests that the farmers' markets, once accessible, will provide fresh fruits and vegetables. By consuming these products, children will lose weight. A measure that would indicate that the program is working would be the number of farmers' markets that spring up within a specified time frame; these are outputs. Outputs are provide the numbers produced and not the impact of the activity. Outputs do not tell us the effect of the program on childhood obesity. However, in the example, the fact that ten new farmers' markets have been created indicates that a program component is working. Stakeholders may be interested in many of the outputs from their programs. Outputs are the most-often assessed results of a program's implementation in the early stages, before outcomes and effects of the program can be measured. Assessing outputs is a means of determining whether the program is being implemented as planned.

The initiative's short-, medium-, and long-term outcomes form another critical component of the evaluation. Outcome questions are concerned not with whether the program is working but with whether it made a difference.

Table 6.1 presents some questions that can appropriately be asked with regard to each logic-model component.

The Program's Objectives

The objectives adopted during the development phase define the activities of the initiative and the expected outcomes and are the basis for developing the evaluation plan and assessing the implementation and effectiveness of a mature program. The evaluation may assess activity objectives such as, "Volunteers from the Regent Gym will provide

TABLE 6.1.   **Identifying Evaluation Questions**

Logic-Model Component	Appropriate Questions
Resources (Inputs)	What funding, personnel, space, or materials were provided for the initiative?
Activities	What training activities were carried out? What educational activities were carried out to inform legislators of the need for new legislation? What activities were undertaken to address an organizational issue that prevented individuals from getting health care? Was the initiative carried out as specified in the protocol? Who is/is not participating in the initiative? How culturally appropriate is the initiative?
Outputs	How many individuals participated? How many items were purchased and used? Were participants satisfied? How many brochures were printed? How many activities were carried out? Were people trained? If yes, how many? Did coalitions form? Were services provided?
Outcomes (Effects)	What knowledge, attitude, skill, and/or behavior changes occurred in the participants who were exposed to the initiative? Were participants of the initiative more or less successful than those who did not participate? What effect did the enactment of the policy have on underage drinking? What are the costs/benefits associated with the program compared with those of similar programs?

information and outreach activities in the community surrounding the Regent Gym for sixty days before the start of the cycling intervention to raise awareness of the importance of exercise for cardiac health." Alternatively, it may decide to assess outcomes such as, "By the end of the three-month intervention, 50 percent of the participants in the Regent Gym cycling intervention will report cycling at least thirty minutes per day." In addition to objectives that serve as benchmarks for the program, stakeholders may identify principles against which the initiative can be appraised. These principles may include social justice and the equitable and ethical distribution of benefits, goods, and services.

Expertise of the Evaluator

Evaluators with a high level of expertise and experience may provide additional insights into the program that lead to added ways of thinking about the evaluation. The expertise of the evaluator and the evaluation team determine the most appropriate evaluation design for conducting the study.

APPROACHES TO SELECTING THE EVALUATION QUESTIONS

The evaluation team must select the research questions that best provide information for decision making and that improve evaluation knowledge and practice. There are many approaches for identifying the research question. One uses a participatory group process and a two-by-two table.

One participatory group process is the *nominal group technique* (Delbecq, Van de Ven, & Gustafson, 1975). A suggested modified nominal group process is as follows:

1. Each member of the stakeholder group makes a list of evaluation questions he or she would like answered.

2. The facilitator asks members of the group in turn to provide one question each to a "master list" on a flip chart or a board that is visible to the whole group. As an evaluation question is added, a show of hands provides a count of how many people included a similar question in their lists. This number is recorded next to the question on the flip chart. The questions on the participants' lists are cancelled as they are accounted for on the master list.

3. The process continues until all members have contributed all the items on their lists that are different from previous questions and all the questions have been crossed off their list.

4. The facilitator reviews the master list with the group and, with the consensus of the group, eliminates or merges questions that appear similar and that ask fundamentally the same question.

The final list sets the stage for deciding on the final set of questions. A traditional two-by-two table can be used to sort the questions and identify priorities. If the evaluation is to be useful and the results utilized, questions that are of primary

FIGURE 6.3.   *Two-by-Two Table*

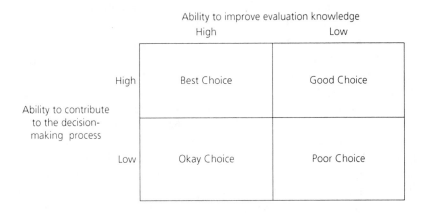

Ability to improve evaluation knowledge

	High	Low
High	Best Choice	Good Choice
Low	Okay Choice	Poor Choice

Ability to contribute to the decision-making process

importance to the person(s) requesting the evaluation or to other stakeholders must be answered.

As shown in Figure 6.3, each evaluation question is reviewed and placed in the appropriate box. If the evaluation team considers that the question will have a high impact in its ability to contribute to the decision-making process and to improve evaluation knowledge, the question is put into the quadrant labeled "best choice." Another question that might have a high impact in contributing to decision making but does not improve evaluation knowledge overall goes in the "good choice" box. This process continues until all the questions are placed. Once this process is complete, the questions in the "best choice" and "good choice" quadrants are the most valuable because evaluation is primarily about the initiative being assessed and evaluation must contribute to decision making. Research-oriented evaluations may want to answer questions in the "okay choice" quadrant. Questions that fall into the "poor choice" quadrant may not warrant time or resources as they neither improve knowledge overall or contribute to decision making.

TYPES OF EVALUATIONS

Once this selection process is complete, a review of the questions that meet the criteria for the evaluation will determine the focus of the evaluation. If the selection process led to questions that were focused primarily on understanding the implementation of the program or policy initiative, then a process evaluation is the appropriate approach. If the selection process led to the identification of questions about the effectiveness of a program that is already stable, then an outcome evaluation is appropriate.

In process evaluation the focus is on the implementation of the initiative at any stage of the program. A process evaluation focuses on the hows and whys of a program and gets at the question, What works? It may also be used to get at the question, How can the program improve what it does? It is then more appropriately called a formative evaluation (Daponte, 2008). A well-conducted process evaluation precedes an outcome evaluation. Determining the level and scope of the initiative's implementation will provide information with regard to why the program is effective and provide the context for an outcome evaluation.

An outcome evaluation assesses the effectiveness of the fully implemented and stabilized initiative and measures the extent to which the initiative made a difference to those who were exposed to it. It addresses concerns that were identified in the needs assessment. An outcome evaluation may ask questions such as, Did participants in the program increase their knowledge, self-care, or utilization of services? Did the community improve access to services? Did the organizations provide needed services for their patients? Did the public policies instituted to reduce the risk of disease, disability, or death make a difference? Did the program have an effect on reducing greenhouse gases? The evaluation may also ask, What were the costs and benefits associated with conducting the intervention? Was the outcome of the program worth the investment?

Yet another approach is to conduct an impact evaluation in order to assess broad changes in quality of life that occur at the local, state, and national levels. An impact evaluation may ask questions such as, Did the programs that were instituted in this community make a difference in the incidence, prevalence, or rates of disease? Did the quality of life of the residents improve? This book focuses primarily on process and outcome evaluation.

PROCESS EVALUATION

Process evaluation is an ongoing check of the implementation of an initiative; it provides information on the extent to which the program is being implemented as planned (Stufflebeam & Shinkfield, 2007). It may assess the context, the reach, the dosage, or intensity of the initiative and the fidelity with which it is delivered. Process evaluation assesses the initiative at the level of resources/inputs and outputs and determines the effectiveness of the administrative functions of the program. It provides information that is used to improve intervention activities and operations. It documents whether the initiative is meeting participants' needs; it identifies any barriers to program implementation; and it looks at participation levels and satisfaction. It asks these questions:

- Is the program/intervention being implemented according to the plan that was laid out before the program started?

- What type, quantity, and quality of services are being provided and to whom?

- What are the products of the program's implementation?

Fundamentally, process evaluation assesses "what works" and establishes the initiative's ability or inability to achieve its outcome objectives. It monitors whether the intervention is being delivered with fidelity. Determining what works for changing policy in a community through an initiative of a statewide community-based organization may lead to a list of questions such as:

- Who are the participants in advocating for, developing, and changing the policy?

- What human, financial, and material resources were provided and used?

- What educational and advocacy activities were carried out?

- Were all the components of the plan implemented? If not, why not?

- What was the level of implementation of the initiative?

- How extensive was the intervention?

- What methods were used to recruit participants? When and how many were used?

- What coalitions were formed?

- What materials were developed?

- What training was provided or received?

- Are the resources provided for this program adequate?

- Are the data-collection tools appropriate for assessing program outcomes?

- Do preliminary findings indicate that the intervention is likely to produce the anticipated outcomes?

Answering a process question requires the evaluation team to determine whether the initiative is being implemented according to plan and whether the intended individuals are participating.

Considerations in whether to conduct process research include:

- The feasibility of the evaluation based on the available resources

- The budget, expertise, and experience of the evaluation team

- Time available for the evaluation process

- Access to and availability of administrative and participant data

- Availability of other data and ability to collect them

Determining Resources, Processes, and Outputs

A process evaluation generally measures resources, activities, and outputs as they pertain to the implementation of the initiative.

Assessing the Resources In answering the question, What human, financial and material resources were provided and used by the initiative?, the components that are assessed will include:

- Funding levels and distribution of financing

- Resources available and utilized for delivering the initiative

- Number and qualifications of staff and others implementing the program

- Quality of the curriculum used for training those delivering the program and for program participants

Assessing the Processes   In answering the questions, Was the initiative implemented as described in the plan? and How well was the program implemented?, the components that are assessed will include:

- Implementation of components of the initiative

- Intensity and reach of activities

- Participation of target population

- Staffing for program activities

- Training

Assessing the Outputs   Outputs are the specific products that result from the initiative. Components for assessing the outputs of a program will include:

- Materials developed

- Services provided

- People trained

- Plans put into operation

The outputs of the initiative are the products of the initiative, so to assess the products we have to know what the initiative was intended to produce. We get this information from the description of the program and from a well-developed and complete logic model. Another source is the activity objectives. Example: By January 2012, twenty-five youth ages eighteen to twenty-five will have access to well-supervised rock-climbing trainings. The activity is the twenty-five trainings, and the product is trained youth. Information on outputs may also be contained in other project documents.

Once we know what was expected from the project documents or from our knowledge of the programs, the next task is to determine whether the outputs exist. In the rock-climbing example, the specific outputs would be

- the number, gender, and race/ethnicity of the trained youth

- the level of participation in the training

- the satisfaction of the youth with the training program

- unanticipated outputs from the training that may have been observed

- the type and level of supervision

Indicators

Indicators are the quantitative or qualitative variables that allow the changes that occur as a result of an intervention to be measured. Indicators show whether the intended results are achieved. They are objectively verifiable and can be assessed repeatedly. One indicator that the rock-climbing training was carried out is the signature of each person who attended on a sign-in sheet. Or each person might be required to complete a satisfaction survey with indicators of attendance and satisfaction. Quantitative indicators measure changes in numerical values; qualitative indicators measure changes that are less well defined but that are agreed to by the stakeholders as measures of success. Indicators are the standards against which performance of the initiative is measured.

Because a large part of the responsibility in process evaluation is process monitoring and documenting the initiative's day-to-day activities and expenditures in a consistent manner, data may be collected by visiting and observing activities and reviewing documents like work plans and minutes from meetings (Stufflebeam & Shinkfield, 2007). Indicators that the event occurred can be found in logs, surveys, individual interviews, and focus groups; discussions with program staff and beneficiaries could be used to complement these indicators. Numerical indicators that show a change has occurred can be plotted in a bar graph, as in Figure 6.4.

OUTCOME EVALUATION

Outcome evaluations ask, Did the initiative make a difference to those who were exposed to it? They assess the expected effects as well as the unexpected effects of the program. They assess whether there was a change in the indicators and determine

FIGURE 6.4.   *Performance of the Indicator Following an Intervention*

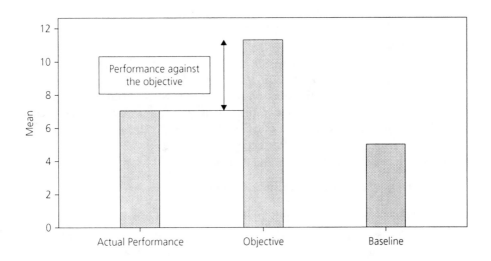

whether the change was caused by the program. Unlike a process evaluation, which is carried out throughout the program, outcome evaluations are carried out after the program is stable and the initiative is expected to have had an effect that is measurable. Carrying out an effective outcome evaluation requires that baseline data be collected for each participant and each indicator. Baseline data are collected prior to implementing the initiative. As in conducting a process evaluation, carrying out an outcome evaluation requires knowledge of how to reach the population, the resources for carrying out the evaluation, the expertise available, and the time line.

Outcome evaluation questions may include:

- Did participants' level of knowledge or awareness change with regard to the program focus?

- What percentage of participants increased their use of a product for the prevention of a disease or disability?

- What percentage of participants reduced their exposure to disease or disability?

- Did the reduction of pollutants in the air reduce the rates of asthma among children one to five years old?

- Did a policy that was aimed at reducing the incidence of violence in a local community have any effect on violence among youth eighteen to twenty-five years old?

- Did an intervention to reduce attacks on the elderly result in fewer seniors with life-threatening injuries over a twelve-month period?

- What were the costs of the initiative relative to the benefits?

As described previously in this chapter, a two-by-two table may be used to identify the questions that are important for the evaluation.

Measuring Concepts and Constructs

Outcome evaluation often uses surveys, individual interviews, focus groups, and observations to assess concepts and constructs that can be difficult to measure. The process of specifying the indicator for measurement involves putting the concepts fully into operation and then deciding on the best means for determining their existence within the sample being studied. Either qualitative or quantitative data-collection approaches can be used. Such measurement requires the specification of one or a number of indicators of the presence or absence of the phenomenon. For example, access to care could be measured at one or more domains:

- Individual level (knowledge, attitude, practices)

- Interpersonal level (peer or family influences)

- Community level (jobs and transportation and their influence on utilization)

- Organizational level (organizational norms, practices, and services that influence an individual's ability to access services within the institution)

- Public-policy level (laws and policies that influence utilization of services by members of the community)

The approach that is adopted in the measurement of access to health care allows for different conclusions to be drawn. Incorporating more than one domain allows for a comprehensive view of issues and the root causes that affect access; measuring access only at the individual level leads to a more restricted view, and hence there are fewer indicators to measure.

Once the measure has been fully conceptualized and the indicator has been specified, decisions can be made about the approach to measurement. The conceptualization of a measurement and the choice of an indicator may differ from one researcher to another and are often influenced by the researcher's discipline and the available knowledge about the concept. The team of evaluators discusses measurement issues for the evaluation and relies on both their expertise and existing research and practice to develop the data-collection instruments.

If the outcome being measured is the extent to which an enacted policy is affecting access to health care, the indicators could be utilization patterns and the number of registered clients. Measurements of these indicators should be made before and after the policy enactment and implementation. Determining such outcomes as change in access to health care requires the use of experimental or quasi-experimental evaluation research designs.

Evaluation Research Designs

To determine outcomes and test the efficacy of an intervention, a rigorous research design using a control or comparison group may be required to produce defensible conclusions. In answering questions related to causation and testing the underlying assumption that the initiative caused the outcome, the beneficiaries of the program are compared with themselves before and after the program or to a similar sample of people who did not participate in the initiative.

Assessing outcomes may include assessing knowledge, attitudes, behaviors, frequency, and the existence or nonexistence of an indicator. Or it may involve using biological or chemical markers in the participants or the environment to determine, for example, whether a test result changes from negative to positive, whether blood pressure rises or falls, or whether hemoglobin A1c levels have changed.

Determining whether the initiative made a difference requires the use of experimental or quasi-experimental evaluation designs. In an experimental research design, groups are created by randomly assigning individuals to the intervention or the control group. However, in public health quasi-experimental designs are considered more appropriate than experimental designs for assessing the impact of initiatives on population samples and populations at large. Quasi-experimental research designs use non randomly assigned groups for comparison.

Many evaluations rely on less rigorous designs that have neither a baseline nor a comparison or control group. These are often called *observational* or *nonexperimental* designs. These evaluations are less time consuming, require fewer resources, and require less expertise than more rigorous designs, but without a baseline, a comparison group, or a control group little can be said about the effectiveness of the intervention. In the simplest designs the intervention is tested in a single after-intervention-only assessment with one data point. An improved design to assess the effect of the initiative is comparing the population sample before and after the initiative in a single-sample pre/post–test design. This chapter provides a brief overview of the commonly used designs for conducting less involved and less complicated evaluations. Detailed explanations of evaluation design may be found in other texts (for example, Cook & Campbell, 1979).

Single-Sample Designs   In a single-sample design, there is no comparison group, and measurements are taken only of the group that is exposed to or that experiences the initiative. Measurements may be taken either after the exposure in a post-only design or before and after in the improved pre/post design. The assessments may be conducted using either qualitative or quantitative measures.

Post-only: $X \, O_1$

Pre/post: $O_1 \, X \, O_2$

The designs are represented by notations that show the intervention as X and the measurement of the change that is observed or measured as O.

The pre/post intervention design allows a comparison of baseline data to postintervention data with the assumption that only the initiative could have changed the data. If O_1 is significantly different from O_2 and there were not likely to have been any other influences on the beneficiaries of the intervention, the initiative might have produced the change.

These are designs that may be familiar, and you have probably used them to evaluate workshops and training, but they are usually ineffective for assessing whether the intervention caused any significant outcomes, especially in uncontrolled environments.

The satisfaction gained from participating in an intervention would be more appropriately measured in a post-only design, while knowledge gained or the effect of a policy change is more appropriately measured in pre/post designs. In general the design used to assess the outcome is dependent on the research question, the most appropriate approach to answer the question, and the expertise and preferences of the evaluator and the evaluation team. The other factor that determines whether a pre/post design can be used is the ability to collect the data before the intervention and after the intervention.

Let us look at a specific example. The research question is, Did the participants in the one-day workshop on policy advocacy improve their knowledge of strategies for improving children's utilization of dental care? Using the pre/post design, this question can be answered by conducting a survey before and after the policy workshop using a combination of quantitative and qualitative measures. Questions in the survey should be limited to information provided during the workshop in order to determine whether the changes in scores were a result of participating in the workshop and relate to the content provided in the workshop. The difference between the baseline data (O_1) and the posttest data (O_2) is the change that occurred in the knowledge levels of participants (Figure 6.5).

This is a very controlled environment, so it is relatively easy to tell that participants increased their learning between coming into the workshop and completing the workshop. However, imagine trying to use the pre/post design in a large community; it would be impossible to draw any meaningful conclusions in such an uncontrolled environment. But there are other ways to design a study that increase confidence in the results.

Time-Series Design A single-group design with multiple measures is an improvement over the single-group design just described. A time-series design takes the measurements over an extended period to determine whether intervention effects are sustained. Using a time-series design may involve the use of historical or secondary data for some or all of the measurement points. A significant limitation of these simple designs is they do little to address threats to internal validity, as discussed later in this chapter.

Comparison-Group Designs Adding a comparison group improves the single-sample design. A comparison group is as similar as possible to the intervention group, but the comparison group does not receive the intervention. Measurements are taken of the individual, group, or community exposed to the intervention and the comparison

FIGURE 6.5. *Mean Scores Before and After an Intervention*

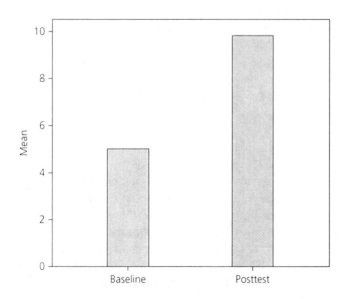

Post-only: $X\ O_1\ O_2\ O_3\ O_4\ O_5$

Pre/post: $O_1\ O_2\ O_3\ O_4\ O_5\ X\ O_6\ O_7\ O_8\ O_9\ O_{10}$

individual, group, or community at the same time. These designs address many but not all of the threats to internal validity, as described later in this chapter. The following diagram reflects the changes to the design notation.

	Post-only	Pre/post
Intervention group	$X\ O_1$	$O_1\ X\ O_2$
Comparison group	O_1	$O_1\ \ O_2$

Note that the comparison group does not receive the intervention (X).

To give an example, let us assume Antoinette's team is assessing a policy-information workshop at a public health facility that has sixty staff members. Two groups of twenty receive the training. The first group can use the second group as its comparison group, with the second group receiving the intervention later. A third group of twenty, who are not exposed to the contents of the workshop, can serve as the comparison group for the second group. The third group may attend a training after the first two workshops are completed, but because that group is not part of the research study, it does not need a comparison group, and no data need be collected. Providing the training to the third group is dependent on resources, but doing so addresses the issue of fairness.

Time-Series Designs with a Comparison Group   A comparison group can be incorporated into a time-series, pre/post design. As described above, the groups must be similar. Note also that the comparison group does not receive the intervention.

	Post-only	Pre/post
Intervention group	$X\ O_1\ O_2\ O_3\ O_4\ O_5$	$O_1\ O_2\ O_3\ O_4\ O_5\ X\ O_6\ O_7\ O_8\ O_9\ O_{10}$
Comparison group	$O_1\ O_2\ O_3\ O_4\ O_5$	$O_1\ O_2\ O_3\ O_4\ O_5\ \ \ O_6\ O_7\ O_8\ O_9\ O_{10}$

Efficiency Assessments

Cost-benefit or cost-effectiveness analyses of a public health initiative assess the efficiency of a program. Such analyses complement outcome assessments and can be used only after the program's outcomes are attained. Cost-benefit analysis requires recording all direct and indirect costs of inputs as well as estimates of all tangible and intangible benefits of the initiative. Cost-effectiveness analysis allows the selection of one intervention over another (Russell, Siegal, Daniels, Gold, Luce & Mandelblatt, 1997). All the costs and benefits are specified in monetary terms, although doing so can prove difficult. Imagine trying to give a value to the multiple tangible and intangible benefits of a child-care program!

Data for assessing the efficiency of an initiative must be gathered from all units participating in the initiative. These cost-related data can be gathered from organizational records and receipts from staff, volunteers, and other stakeholders:

- Administrative expenditures include salaries, incentives, and travel expenses of personnel; costs for office space, utilities, and office supplies; costs of running the office—for example, photocopying expenses; office-maintenance costs, such as outlays for cleaning, repairs, insurance, and equipment.

- Direct costs associated with initiative implementation include participant stipends; transportation reimbursements; costs for child care; cost of supplies, such as games, food, books; rent for space/venue; cost of amenities; cost of equipment; costs associated with instituting a policy; costs to the beneficiaries of the initiative of participating in the intervention or of adopting a policy.

- Unintended costs associated with initiative implementation are the unexpected costs engendered by a new initiative (program or policy).

The benefits-related data may be more difficult than the cost data to obtain. They include such items as the value of play areas for children, lives saved, improved health status, or quality of life. Benefits may also be the cost savings that accrue in the long term.

Cost-benefit and cost-effectiveness analyses require skills that may not be available on the evaluation team. Accounting and economics experts may be needed to support this kind of evaluation.

Internal and External Validity

Internal Validity   *Internal validity* is the extent to which an effect that is observed was caused by a systematically planned intervention (Cook & Campbell, 1979) and does not occur in the absence of the intervention.

In assessing the outcomes of an intervention in an experimental or quasi-experimental evaluation research design, we would like to conclude that the result that occurs in the intervention group does not appear in the control or comparison group. We assume that the difference is real and is not due to random or systematic error. When we draw this conclusion correctly, we can claim that the intervention caused the outcomes we observed.

However, when we draw this conclusion erroneously and conclude that the intervention had an impact on the intervention group and not the control or comparison group when, in fact, the intervention group and the control group did not differ, then we have a *Type I error*. When we draw the conclusion also erroneously that the intervention had no impact when in fact it did and the results for the intervention group should have been different from the results for the control or comparison group, then we have a *Type II error*.

It is important to consider the multiple factors that may influence the evaluator's ability to conclude that the intervention resulted in the observed changes. The factors that prevent or limit an evaluator's confidence that the initiative caused the effect (outcome) are referred to as threats to (internal) validity. The most frequent threats to validity, which are discussed in detail by Cook and Campbell (1979), are summarized here.

Attrition: A loss of participants in the intervention that is different from the loss that occurs in the initially similar control group results in having different kinds and different numbers of people in the posttest phase.

History: Events that take place outside the intervention may affect the measurement of changes that are due to the program. Such events may result in an inflation of posttest scores.

Instrumentation: Changes occur to the reliability and validity of measurement tools used to assess the effect of the program.

Maturation: Changes in the study participants that are due to natural and physiological development take place over time and are not necessarily caused by the program. Such natural changes may occur in children and in the elderly.

Regression: When study participants are selected on the basis of high or low baseline scores, the results of the testing will show they regress toward the population mean. High scorers will show lower scores in the posttest, and low scorers will show higher scores.

Selection: Differences in the intervention and the comparison group occur when people self-select into the groups or when people drop out of the groups disproportionately. The result is that those who stay may be likely to succeed with or without the program

Statistical conclusion: The sample size is too small to show the effect or the measurement instruments are unstable and unlikely to measure true changes because of high standard-error estimates. Other statistical-conclusion threats include violated assumptions of statistical tests and the likelihood of concluding that there is covariance when there is not, as in Type 1 errors. "Fishing" occurs when multiple comparisons are run during a statistical analysis without recognizing that the results may be significantly different just by chance.

Testing: Changes that occur to the study participants when a test that is given before the intervention may affect the results when the test is given again after the intervention in pre/post designs. The threat may be due to participants' familiarity with the test items and their error responses if they remember them.

The evaluation designs that contain single sample pre/post measurements and those utilizing comparisons groups address the threats to validity to a lesser or greater extent. The single-group post-only design is the least likely to minimize threats to internal validity, while experimental evaluation designs using randomly assigned controls and intervention groups and communities are the most likely to minimize these threats, and therefore they allow the most certainty that the intervention caused the changes that occurred in the beneficiaries. In a quasi-experimental design many of the threats to validity are addressed also, but they may require additional measures to ensure the same level of confidence that randomly assigned control groups provide. Measures include using matching and randomly selected groups (not individuals) in a model that promises a delayed intervention.

Additional threats to internal validity take place that are not minimized by using randomized samples:

- *Diffusion* or *imitation* occurs when the information intended for the treatment group is obtained by the control group; the difference between the treatment and control group is thereby narrowed.

- *Compensatory equalization* occurs when the control group is provided with or obtains an alternative intervention that results in narrowing the differences between the treatment group and the control group.

- *Compensatory rivalry* occurs when the control group works hard to rival the intervention group to improve their outcomes; such rivalry minimizes the differences between groups (Cook & Campbell, 1979).

External Validity *External validity* is the extent to which an observed effect (outcome) can be generalized to other times, settings, and populations (Cook & Campbell, 1979). The larger and more heterogeneous the sample that participates in an intervention that is found to be internally valid, the more likely it is that the outcome is generalizable. One of the most important threats to external validity is selection bias, which may be inherent in the selection of the participants or which may occur in the loss of participants resulting from attrition. The effect in either case is a more homogenous and biased sample than would otherwise exist.

SUMMARY

- Evaluation questions are best selected through a participatory process involving the evaluators and the stakeholders. Utilizing a two-by-two table allows the group to arrive at a set of appropriate evaluation questions.

- Process evaluation questions ask whether the program was implemented as planned. They assess the initiative at the level of resources, inputs, and outputs, including the administrative functions of the program.

- In assessing efficiency, the perspectives from which the costs and benefits may be assessed are participants, program sponsors, and overall costs to society, the societal costs being the most difficult to value monetarily.

(Continued)

(Continued)

▪ In determining outcomes and the efficacy of an intervention, a rigorous research design using a control or comparison group may be required to produce defensible conclusions.

▪ Internal validity describes a causal relationship; external validity describes the generalizability of the intervention across time, people, and places. A Type I error occurs when it is erroneously assumed that the intervention caused the outcome. A Type II error occurs when it is erroneously found that the intervention did not have an effect on the outcome.

DISCUSSION QUESTIONS AND ACTIVITIES

1. Identify a program of your choice and develop a logic model. Write twenty questions that correspond to the components in the logic model. Divide the set of questions into process and outcome evaluation questions. Given the number of each, what kind of evaluation would most likely be conducted?

2. Think of a concept you would like to understand. Fully conceptualize it and identify the variables that you would need to assess to get at this concept. Conduct a literature review of the concept. How has it been assessed by other researchers?

3. Enumerate the threats to internal validity. To what extent do the different evaluation designs minimize these threats?

KEY TERMS

attrition threats to internal validity
experimental design
external validity
fidelity
history threats to internal validity
implementation
indicator
instrumentation threats to internal validity
internal validity
maturation threats to internal validity

observational/nonexperimental design
outcome evaluation
process evaluation
quasi-experimental design
regression threats to internal validity
selection
statistical-conclusion threats to internal validity
testing threats to internal validity
Type I error
Type II error

CHAPTER

7

COLLECTING THE DATA

QUANTITATIVE

LEARNING OBJECTIVES

- Identify and describe data-collection approaches for quantitative research.
- Explain how to ascertain reliability and validity in quantitative research.
- Describe the functions of an Institutional Review Board.

Answering the research question requires using one of a variety of approaches, all of which require the collection of data. Data collection for process evaluation requires reviewing financial statements, audit reports, travel documents, invoices, contracts, administrative logs, participation logs, sign-in and activity sheets, training logs, meeting notes, and surveys. Data collection for outcome evaluation requires a number of specific and deliberate data-collection steps and activities at the beginning, during, and at the end of the initiative; such data collection involves quantitative combined with qualitative approaches.

The second step of the Participatory Model for Evaluation is to collect the data (see Figure 7.1). This and the next chapter focus on collecting and analyzing quantitative data to answer the research questions in either process or outcome evaluation. Applying the Community-Based Participatory Research principles to quantitative data collection requires paying particular attention to the participation of stakeholders in the conceptualization, development, and implementation of the methods (Keiffer, Salabarria-Pena, Odoms-Young, Willis, Baber, & Gusman, 2005; Schulz, Zenk, Kannan, Israel, Koch, & Stokes, 2005).

CHOOSING A DATA-COLLECTION APPROACH

In both quantitative and qualitative data collection, the approaches used to collect primary data should be the most appropriate for answering the research question and should always be based on the needs of the project. The data collection for a simple

FIGURE 7.1.   *The Participatory Framework for Evaluation: Collect the Data*

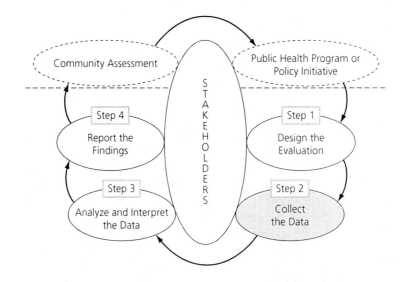

pre/post test necessitates different expertise, training, and approaches than the data collection for a quasi-experimental or experimental design.

The most appropriate approach is the one most likely to provide valid and reliable data. A number of factors influence the credibility of the data that are collected, including whether

- appropriate methods are used

- multiple methods are used

- sources from which the data are collected are reliable

- theoretical frameworks for developing the data-collection instruments are used

- the biases associated with the recruitment of the study participants and the data-collection methods are minimized

- the quality and the quantity of the data collected are sufficient

Important considerations for both quantitative and qualitative research are the characteristics of the study participants, which may influence the approach that is selected. The approach selected should also ensure the right of the individual to respect and fair treatment. Consideration must be given to respondents'

- culture and cultural values

- educational levels and preferences

- age, gender, race/ethnicity

- accessibility and availability

- access to computer technology

- access to telephones

- right to refuse to participate

The availability of resources also influences the type and duration of the monitoring and the type and quality of the conclusions. The better the quality of the data, the more valid the conclusions. Factors that influence the quality and the quantity of the data include:

- Appropriate and effective staff support

- Language capabilities for conducting culturally sensitive interactions and interviews

- Logistics support for project management and data collection

- Time allocated for completing the study

- Technology capability for data collection and analysis

- Availability of stipends and incentives

- Possibilities for translating instruments, transcribing interviews, and entering, coding, and analyzing data)

USING SURVEYS

Surveys are the most often used data-collection tool for quantitative research designed to collect information from those who experience or have a personal insight into the issue being assessed. Individuals may be members of the community and affected by the problem, as in health assessments, or may be providers of the services. Key informants, who see the problem from their own vantage point but have considerable insight, may also be surveyed.

Using surveys as a data-collection method has several advantages:

- Constructing items for a valid and reliable survey can be a difficult and time-consuming exercise; but once the items are developed, they may be used over and over again for similar projects.

- Surveys are relatively easy to administer; they collect a large amount of data in a relatively short period of time.

- Surveys can be evaluated for reliability and validity.

- Surveys lend themselves easily to communitywide data-collection efforts.

- Written surveys can be administered in groups or individually, by mail, face to face, by telephone or electronically.

- Surveys are generally less expensive to administer than other research instruments.

There are several considerations in opting to conduct surveys:

- Surveys collect large amounts of data that provide some information but often leave the researcher asking, Why or So what?

- Surveys have to be just the right length, long enough to measure the concepts accurately and ensure stability of the measure, but short enough to be completed fully and not burden the respondent unduly.

- The time or expertise it takes to develop a reliable and valid survey instrument may not be available. Survey administration can take a long time to complete as respondents may not respond to a request to complete it face to face, open their mail for a mail-in survey, answer the telephone, or respond to an e-mail request. Getting the survey completed may take several attempts at contacting the potential respondents through reminder post cards or multiple phone calls and e-mails spread over an extended period.

Surveys may be used to collect information in a community assessment, as baseline data before or at the start of an initiative, and in assessing the process or outcomes of an intervention. Like all other measurement tools, they can be used in any of the evaluation research designs. Often they are used when there is no specific research design.

Surveys require a considerable amount of skill to develop and analyze. One of my students had this to say about the process: "Although it could take multiple hours and many drafts [to develop] your survey or questionnaire, it is best to put the time in[to] creating it, and . . . this will make the remainder of the process go a lot smoother."

Maximizing the potential for the survey to provide the best information requires engaging diverse stakeholders in the conceptualization of the survey, the identification of specific survey areas and items, the selection of survey language and wording, and the approaches to survey administration (Israel et al., 2005, p. 108).

In addition, a variety of activities can improve survey instruments, including:

- Using expert panels to assure appropriate and complete understanding of the concept being measured

- Using a pilot test with the potential study population to ensure understanding of the survey items

- Incorporating tests of validity and reliability

- Providing appropriate and adequate training to the people collecting the data

- Partnering with trained and experienced statisticians or biostatisticians to make sample-size calculations, determine appropriate formats, and analyze data

If resources are available and it is appropriate to develop web-based surveys, a variety of survey-development tools are available to support this process. These online tools include SurveyMonkey® and Zommerang®. The online tools provide easy-to-follow directions and formatting options. In addition, for computer-distributed surveys they may also offer appropriate distribution options. Once the surveys are completed and returned the tools offer some simple data-analysis options and the opportunity to download the participant data into other data-analysis software such as Microsoft Excel® and SPSS®, a statistical data-mining and analysis software for analyzing quantitative data.

Administering Surveys

Surveys may be completed by self-administration, in face-to-face or telephone interviews, or through online distribution either directly on the web or via e-mail. Questionnaires are most valuable for collecting data from a large number of people. Considerations in the selection of the method include the type of information required, the population to be surveyed, and the financial resources, human resources, and time available.

The type of information that is required often determines the approach to survey administration. The more sensitive the information, the less likely some individuals are to want to discuss it with another person, so an interviewer-facilitated survey may be less successful than a self-administered survey. Face-to-face interviews may be appropriate with less-sensitive questions. Obtaining information through interviews requires the interviewer to be tactful and to build rapport with the interviewee. Both open-ended and closed-ended questions may be used in surveys conducted face-to-face or by telephone; getting information from open-ended questions is less successful in a self-administered format. Telephone interviews tend to have less missing data and fewer "don't know" responses than self-administered surveys (Feveile, Olsen, & Hugh, 2007), although building rapport for a good telephone interview may be difficult. A face-to-face interview will likely produce more valid information than a self-completed survey in populations with low reading levels.

The resources available for the distribution of surveys or to conduct interviewer-facilitated surveys may control the approach that is selected. Face-to-face meetings require additional time, training, and travel. Mail-distributed surveys incur initial postage costs and postage for follow-up and reminder post cards. Although the cost of distributing surveys by e-mail is low, the likelihood of having wrong e-mail addresses is high. Utilizing telephones may require high tolls for long-distance calls.

The most appropriate method for administering surveys is often based on the population that the survey is intended to reach. Participants who do not have telephones cannot be reached with a survey using this technology; a web-based survey cannot reach somebody who neither has nor uses a computer.

The channel that is used for survey distribution influences the response rate and how quickly the study can be completed. Mail-distributed surveys require an initial notification of the survey's arrival by letter or post card and multiple reminders, which include further mailing or telephone calls to request the survey's completion. Recent access to computer technology has made e-mails and web-based computer distribution an option, but access to the various technologies may affect survey distribution and completion.

Ensuring That Data Are Valid and Reliable

When survey instruments are developed they are subjected to a variety of procedures to increase both their validity and reliability. Validity and reliability are standards for measurements, and they thus dictate collection processes. Validity is the extent to which a measure assesses the underlying concept that it claims to measure. Reliability refers to the consistency of the measure when it is applied repeatedly. Reliability is assessed using internal consistency, split-halves, and retest methodologies (Carmines & Zeller, 1979).

Although reliability and validity are assessed separately, there is a relationship between the two that is worth remembering. For an instrument to be reliable, it must also be valid, but it can be valid without being reliable. So it is important in evaluation to ensure that any tool that is used to measure a concept, a construct, or an outcome is valid.

Validity Validity concerns the degree to which scores that are achieved reflect the underlying construct. Three types of validity are generally associated with instrument development: construct validity, content validity, and criterion validity (Carmines & Zeller, 1979).

Construct validity is the extent to which the measure is theoretically sound and correlates with the theorized construct. It measures phenomena that can be observed that reflect the underlying concepts. *Content validity* assesses the extent to which the items in an instrument are well defined and represent all the facets of a given construct. Experts may be used during the instrument-development phase to assess the accuracy of the items that are selected to measure the variable of interest. A literature review or qualitative research may also provide information to improve conceptualization and understanding of the variables and their impact on the measurement. *Criterion validity* describes the concurrence of the item or scale with a previously assigned "gold standard" that confirms its predictive value (Carmines & Zeller, 1979).

Reliability When an instrument is developed, it is assessed for its stability in order to determine the level of random error that may be interfering with true measurement of the variable. Any error variability causes an underestimation or overestimation of the true measurement making the assessment unreliable. This variability is measured using a reliability coefficient that is at 1.0 when no error exists.

A range of approaches can be used to assess the extent to which there is variability in the collection and interpretation of the data. Intrarater reliability assesses the extent to which the individual changes with each successive assessment. Interrater reliability measures the differences between two persons assessing the same situation or the same data. Cohen's kappa (Cohen, 1960) is the statistical test generally used to assess reliability using nominal or ordinal data.

Internal consistency is a measure of correlations across given items in a test (Carmines & Zeller, 1979). Cronbach's alpha assesses the correlation among the total number of items on the scale and the extent to which they assess the same underlying concept (Windsor, Clark, Boyd, & Goodman, 2004). An instrument with a high internal-consistency coefficient has an alpha ≤ 1.0. An acceptable range for psychometric analysis of an instrument is ≥ 0.65 to ≤ 0.90.

Test-retest assessment measures reliability by using the same test and administering it two different times with the same sample. To increase the validity of this test, the repeat test must be conducted within a short period of time and must record a Cohen's kappa of ≥ 0.80 (Windsor et al., 2004).

Sample-Selection Approach and Sample Size

An accurate definition of the target population and of the inclusion and exclusion criteria for the study participants are critical in any research study. The sample consists of population units, things, organizations, geographical areas, and so forth that have the characteristics of interest to the researcher. It differs from one research study to another and is directly related to the evaluation question. For instance, a study of the relationship between childhood obesity and the intake of vegetables will likely focus on children ages three to twelve, while a study of substance abuse and teen driving may focus on youth fifteen to twenty-one years old. Sampling is the process of selecting a small set/group of units from the target population.

There are two main types of sampling: random/probability and nonrandom/nonprobability. *Random* selection methods are used when the resulting sample has to be representative of the population. Random sampling is used primarily in quantitative studies, such as surveys, because it enables the researcher to generalize the results to the population as a whole. A sampling frame is required that allows for a random selection of participants who are representative of the underlying population being studied. These approaches are used in designing experimental and quasi-experimental designs and include the use of simple, systematic, cluster, or stratified sampling techniques (Shi, 1997).

Nonrandom methods are used primarily when the goal is to explore and reach an understanding about issues that pertain to a specific group of people. Although these methods are convenient for obtaining a sample for study, they rely on having captive audiences or on the particular characteristics of the population. For instance, it is impossible to randomly select a sample from a hidden or hard-to-reach population, such as illegal immigrants, drug addicts, runaway youths. Although the bias in selection of participants is much higher when using nonrandom sampling techniques, the method can still lead to valid statistical conclusions. Nonrandom sampling includes convenience, purposive, and snowball sampling (Shi, 1997). They do not provide samples that are representative of the underlying population and therefore results from them are not generalizable.

Cluster sampling may be used to select a group or participants from a group or entity such as a business, a school, a faith community, a census tract, or a neighborhood. The entire group or location can be selected, or a randomly selected number of participants may be selected to represent the group or the entity.

Probability sampling involves random selection of the participants in the study. It is achieved by selecting names or numbers at random from a list of all potential participants with each having an equal chance to participate.

Systematic sampling is an alternative strategy to probability sampling. It is achieved by selecting names or numbers from a list such as a voting register or a phone book at the same regular interval.

Stratification sampling is achieved when the members from a population group of interest are subdivided into strata and systematically sampled from a list of the population of interest. The sample that is selected is proportional to the size of the population type in the general population.

The sample size for data collection is determined by the research approach, the population selected, the needs of the study, the type of analysis required, the resources and expertise available, and the cost. The size of a random sample or the number of units on which data have to be collected is computed based on several types of information:

- The size of the population—if known

- The amount of error in prediction that can be tolerated, generally 5 percent, yielding a 95 percent confidence that the study results are accurate

- The effect size, or the degree to which the groups in the study differ in the characteristics of interest in the study—for example, how much heavier kids are who do not have at least one intake of vegetables a day than those who do

The larger the sample the more representative it will be and the more power it will have for making accurate and reliable interpretations of the data; but the cost will be higher also. Sample size is generally computed to give the researcher a minimum of 80 percent power to detect a difference between groups, should the difference exist.

In general, the more heterogeneous the population the larger the sample size required for quantitative-research analysis. The sample size is also determined by the number of variables in the study and the number of subgroup analyses that are proposed. If, for example, a survey was conducted as part of a study about workplace injuries at a treatment plant, a larger sample size would be required to understand the factors leading to the injuries if the analysis were conducted to provide subgroup analysis by gender, age, race, or type of occupation.

The sample size for a research study may be calculated based on a formula from a table or calculated using computer programs such as STATA, SAS, or EpiInfo (Shi, 2008). Detailed discussion of this topic may be found in other texts.

Conducting Survey Research

Before a survey can be taken, it must reach the study population. It is important that the distribution method be sensitive to the cultural norms of the population and appropriate for the setting and the study. Participants for a survey may be available in one place, or they may need to be individually recruited. Advertisements to recruit participants may be placed in flyers and other media. People can also be invited to complete a survey contained within an envelope, placed on a web site, attached to an e-mail, or through a telephone call. Recruitment scripts that are included with the surveys distributed by mail, read over the phone, or included in an online solicitation must be developed and approved by a local Institutional Review Board.

Staff must be hired and trained to conduct telephone or face-to-face interviews for data collection. In an empowerment model, such training leaves communities with skills they can use long after the evaluation. Training may include improving facilitation and listening skills but always includes familiarization with the interview guide so that there is little or no change in its delivery from one interview to the next. Consistent delivery increases reliability and minimizes the threat to validity caused by instrumentation.

DESIGNING SURVEY INSTRUMENTS

Survey-Development Process

Before developing a survey the first consideration is, What is the research question and what information does this survey have to elicit? If the answer is not available in existing data and a new survey has to be developed, then the next question is, Is there a survey available that can be adopted or adapted? Answering the second question requires doing a literature search for peer reviewed articles that contain surveys or results of surveys, consulting with colleagues in the same or a similar field, or scanning the internet. In program evaluation, finding the right survey can be difficult because initiatives are unique and have different characteristics, and the needs of the evaluation can be different each time.

Identifying the questions first requires identifying the indicators for the response. This is achieved through the literature review and, in cases where there is little information about the phenomenon, brainstorming with experts in the field or conducting structured focus-group interviews with a sample of the population. Indicators provide the evidence that a change has occurred. Examples of indicators include:

- The percentage of participants reporting an increase in the number of minutes per day of exercise

- The percentage of respondents registering under a newly implemented expansion of eligibility for health insurance

The responses to questions in pre/post surveys that assess the participant's outcome in relation to the activity may be used as indicators.

Identifying existing reliable and valid instruments that serve the purposes of the study or compiling a new instrument using existing valid and reliable items from a variety of sources may be quicker than developing an instrument from scratch. Modified or new instruments should be validated with a sample similar to the study population in a pilot test.

In developing an instrument, it is essential to keep in mind

- the potential respondents for the survey

- the questions and question formats

- the data-analysis needs

Potential Respondents

The persons required to complete a survey are a key consideration. They will determine the language and the reading level of the survey tools. Surveys to solicit information from Spanish-only speakers will have to be written in Spanish or translated into Spanish. By the same token, if reading levels are low, the survey must be developed at a third- to sixth- grade level in the appropriate language. Particular attention is given to developing surveys for children and adults who function at a lower cognitive level and who have less developed conceptual skills; they require more concrete questions. The Flesch-Kincaid Grade Level Readability Formula developed by Rudolph Flesch and John Kincaid may be used to assess the reading level of surveys. It is built into Microsoft Word® and can be accessed through the spelling and grammar function. A survey also should be developed so its length does not burden respondents unduly. Survey developers must balance their need to know against the real-life experiences of the respondents.

Question Formats

Survey instruments may contain closed-ended, open-ended, or multiple-choice questions or questions that provide three- to five-point scales for respondent feedback. Surveys may also ask respondents to match, rank, or compare a set of options.

Babbie (1990) points out that the response categories of closed-ended questions should be exhaustive, including all the possible responses, and should be mutually exclusive. However, because it is often not possible to meet these criteria, respondents can be given the option of writing in their own response by using the "other" category. These answers are coded before data entry to allow for appropriate analysis.

A survey instrument with closed-ended questions expects responses such as yes/no, ranking responses, and other numerical formats. The type of questions also determines the level of understandability of the items and therefore influences the response. Giving a yes/no response may be easier for a low-level reader than selecting a response on a five-point scale of "very unfavorable to very favorable." However, a survey with only yes/no responses provides limited understanding of underlying concepts and limits the variability in the items. In addition, it limits the level of data analysis that can be conducted. It is important to field-test the instrument with persons similar to those in the final audience to determine how well the items are understood and how well they produce the appropriate responses. Table 7.1 provides some sample questions with corresponding response formats.

A useful addition to closed-ended questions in traditional surveys is the use of open-ended questions. Respondents are asked to provide their own answers to the questions. For example, respondents may be asked to explain a response they gave to a closed-ended question. They may be asked a new question such as "What did you experience when you visited the site of the earthquake?" Lines or a text box are provided for answers. Using open-ended questions as part of a survey provides for deeper understanding of the phenomenon, which is usually not achieved from typical survey research. Answers to open-ended questions may be coded before data entry to allow them to be converted to quantitative data.

Data-Analysis Needs

The question format determines the types of data analysis that can be carried out. *Nominal-level data* are the lowest level and allow for a distinction in mutually exclusive

TABLE 7.1.   **Questions and Response Formats**

Questions	Possible Response Types
Do you know about the recent changes in the policy to increase eligibility?	Yes/no
What is your opinion about the following statement: Changes in the policy improved access to health care for residents of my county.	Five-point scale of strongly disagree to strongly agree
The clinic that was opened in your community recently offers the following services [list of services].	Check all that you might use
What is your opinion about the services provided in the newly opened clinic?	Five-point scale of very unfavorable to very favorable
How old are you?	Age in years
Has having the clinic changed the lives of residents of this community?	Yes/No

categories such as gender (male/female) or place of residence (house, apartment, trailer home, boathouse). When just two categories are given (yes/no), the values are dichotomous. Nominal data are used to calculate percentages. *Ordinal-level data* allow rank ordering within the categories and are represented by a number or a scale with no meaning other than the indication of a rank order. Nominal data are used to calculate percentages and can also be used to calculate means. *Interval-level data* have more meaning than ordinal data because the distances between the points have real meaning on a numerical scale. A commonly used example is the temperature scale, where the difference between eighty degrees and ninety degrees is the same ten degrees as the difference between sixty degrees and seventy degrees. *Ratio-level data* provide a true zero; length, height, and age are good examples (Babbie, 1990). Like interval data, means and standard deviations can be calculated from this category of data and used to summarize the data.

Because the type of data collected determines the type of analysis that can be undertaken, the questions must be designed to ensure that the appropriate level of data is collected. For example, if you are interested in having means, then the data must be ordinal, interval, or ratio data. Once the instrument is developed and those data are collected, only limited analyses may be possible if an inappropriate level of data has been used. For this reason, it is important to consult a statistician at the beginning rather than at the end of survey development.

Steps in Creating a Survey Instrument

When the research question is fully conceptualized through a review of the literature or an expert review panel or by conducting focus groups with the intended audience for the survey, you are ready to frame the specific survey questions. The survey questions are developed to reflect the information that is being sought. They have content validity. It is instructive to have content experts review the questions to ensure that they reflect the concepts that are being measured; additional feedback from a statistician can ensure that appropriate question formats are used for the analysis.

When evaluators must develop their own instrument, they can do so by following these steps:

Step 1: State the evaluation research question and define the indicators that reflect the construct of interest.

Step 2: Frame appropriate questions making them as clear and as simple as possible.

Step 3: Order the questions into an instrument that flows smoothly from beginning to end. Consult a statistician as needed to confirm the appropriateness of the response categories for the proposed data analysis.

Step 4: Review the instrument for construct content validity. Does it ask the question it intends to ask, and does it measure the construct fully? Have an expert panel review the instrument.

Step 5: Check the instrument's readability using the Flesch-Kincaid Grade Level Readability Formula built into Microsoft Word® if required to determine the reading level.

Step 6: Pilot-test the draft instrument with individuals or groups similar to the study population.

Step 7: Edit the survey instrument as needed.

Step 8: Prepare the final instrument for use.

An alternative approach to assembling a set of questions for a survey instrument is by reviewing existing surveys in the literature or by contacting colleagues or experts in the field. Using existing valid and reliable surveys or drawing ideas from them saves time. If you take this route, be sure to get permission to use the material or include a reference if it is a publicly available survey.

Once the final set of questions is ready, the draft instrument is compiled into an easy-to-read, logical format complete with instructions for completing the items. Dillman (2000) suggests that difficult and sensitive questions and demographic questions be left to the end. Once the draft survey is reviewed by an expert panel, it is ready for a pilot test. The extensive use of electronic communication such as e-mail and web-based tools makes reviewing by an expert panel and editing questions a more practical and less time-consuming process than it once was.

Additional guidelines for survey development include:

▪ Make items clear, precise, and short so the respondent knows exactly what the question is that your are asking.

▪ Avoid using items that contain more than one question.

▪ Ask only questions that are important to the respondents and that are relevant to answering the research question.

▪ Avoid asking questions in the negative, using words such as *not*.

▪ Ensure that concepts are clearly defined.

▪ Ensure that questions allow for a normal distribution of responses or a fifty/fifty distribution in the case of dichotomous answers.

▪ Use as large a number of answer categories as possible to provide variability in the responses.

▪ Avoid asking questions that result in the respondent responding to the question in a particular way, either negatively or positively. (Babbie, 1990).

PILOT TESTING

Pilot testing an instrument is a chance to determine whether it works under real-life conditions and whether it works well in the population for which it is intended. Conduct the pilot test with a representative number of participants drawn from the same sampling frame as the one used for the study. Participants in the pilot test must be similar to the study participants. Babbie (1990, p. 227) refers to pilot testing as "a miniaturized walk through of the final survey design."

A pilot test provides an opportunity to determine whether the instrument is culturally appropriate, is written at the appropriate reading level, is short enough so as not to burden the respondent, and is written so that the questions are interpreted by the respondents in ways the researchers intended. Conducting the pilot test also provides opportunities to test the flow of the questions and to time the entire procedure, including administering the consent form. It provides data for instrument validity and reliability tests and is a way to solicit feedback. When the pilot test is complete, the surveys are revised and edited as necessary and they are ready to be rolled out.

A pilot test provides information on:

* The clarity of questions

* The clarity of the response items

* Questions that respondents could not answer or chose not to answer

* The clarity of instructions for answering the questions

* Alternative responses that the respondent may provide that are not represented in the survey. Using an "other" category allows for respondents to provide additional possible answers for the final survey (Babbie, 1990)

Another value in conducting a pilot study beyond field testing the survey is to field-test the entire process and test the prediction that the intervention caused the outcome that is observed (hypothesis) (Babbie, 1990).

TRIANGULATION

Evaluators should not be confined to using only one method if the research can be appropriately conducted using a combination of approaches. Using a mixed-method approach and multiple sources of data or varying data-collection methods to cross-check and substantiate findings and increase validity in evaluation research is known as *triangulation*.

Primary and secondary data can be used to answer the same research question; they provide complementary or differing perspectives. Primary-data sources include:

* People directly affected by the problem

* People implementing initiatives and services to address the problem

* People knowledgeable about the problem

* People observing the behaviors or conditions that influence the problem

* Influential members of society such as policymakers and community leaders

Secondary-data sources include existing local, state, and national data bases that provide behavioral, environmental, and health statistics (Shi, 2008).

In addition to using a variety of sources of data, a mix of qualitative and quantitative data-collection approaches may be used to achieve triangulation. A matrix may be used to think through the selection of the most appropriate approaches. The final selection can be based on considerations of appropriateness, expertise, and resources. The planning process can help delineate these factors for decision making.

INSTITUTIONAL REVIEW BOARDS

During the data-collection process, the rights of individuals must be respected and their welfare must be protected. It is also important to protect privacy and confidentiality in data collection and in reporting the results.

Protecting the rights of an individual requires that researchers do not coerce anyone to participate in a study. In addition, participants have the right to know and understand all the research procedures. If they consent to participate they must be treated in a caring, considerate, and respectful way. All their interactions must be kept confidential, and their data must remain anonymous unless they have been notified otherwise.

Specifically, the American Evaluation Association (2008, p. 234) identifies respect for people as a guiding principle for evaluation practice. "Evaluators respect the security, dignity and self worth of respondents, program participants, clients and other evaluation stakeholders and thus should abide by current professional ethics, standards, and regulations regarding confidentiality, informed consent, and potential risk and harms to participants."

An Institutional Review Board (IRB) is a panel of individuals who represent both the research institution and the community. The board reviews research proposals, provides guidelines about informed-consent documents, and ensures that the research does not have the potential to harm research subjects. Requests for IRB review must contain the full research proposal, data-collection instruments, consent forms, recruitment materials and information provided to the study participants.

Consent forms contain a description of the research study and information about risks, the voluntary nature of the study, and the confidentiality of patient information. They specify the benefits of participating and contact information for an independent institutional representative whom the study participants can get in touch with if necessary. Informed-consent forms must be read by or read to the participant and signed by both the participant and the researcher. Consenting to participation in a research study is also required to be culturally appropriate. Alternative approaches must be sought when necessary. Information provided to the participant in the consent form includes how confidentiality and anonymity of respondents' identity and responses will be maintained.

Informed-consent forms should include the following elements:

▩ The purposes of the research

▩ The expected duration of the subject's participation

▩ The number of people in the study

▩ A description of the procedures

▩ A description of any foreseeable risks or discomforts to the subject

▩ A description of the benefits

▩ An assurance that records will be confidential

- A statement that participation is voluntary

- A description of the compensation provided

- Contact information

Members of research teams are required to complete training on the protection of human subjects and to be familiar with the Health Insurance Portability Act guidelines. See IRB guidelines for your institution for further information.

STAKEHOLDER INVOLVEMENT

Stakeholders provide insight into ensuring the data collected are both reliable and valid. They provide information on the methods that are most appropriate for their community. They may facilitate the data-collection process and collect the data. Stakeholder participation is critical for ensuring that the sample population is knowledgeable about the study and is willing to participate. In small communities previous knowledge of a research activity will often facilitate or hinder data collection. Information about the evaluation can be provided in community meetings and in the print and electronic media. It is important that the potential respondents understand the value of participating in the study.

In Community-Based Participatory Research, members of the community may be trained to collect the data. In many communities this may serve as an advantage as they already have knowledge of the community and an understanding of the issues. As in all well-designed research studies, it is important to minimize the risk of bias in the data collection and the threat to validity known as instrumentation, so adequate training of enumerators and facilitators is critical. It is also important to understand that members of the community may not be the most appropriate people to collect sensitive and personal information. A balance must be struck between using members of the community and collecting valid and reliable data. In some cases using outsiders as data collectors may be preferable. A conversation with the stakeholders may help clarify any issues that arise in the process of data collection.

SUMMARY

- The validity of the evaluation relies on the sample characteristics, the research methodology itself, and its cultural appropriateness.

- Answering the question involves using an appropriate mix of data that are gathered from and about the people who benefit, who provide the goods and services, or who are somehow influenced or affected by the initiative.

- The selection of the method for data collection and data analysis depends on the research approach that is adopted, the expertise and skills of the evaluator, the resources available for the evaluation, and the costs.

(Continued)

(Continued)

▨ Surveys developed to collect quantitative data for evaluation may be administered by a variety of methods that must be sensitive to the context, the population, the type of data, and the type of analysis needed.

▨ Quantitative and qualitative data are both appropriate methods for collecting data to answer an evaluation question; together they provide scope and depth to the findings. Using both primary and secondary data is also useful in providing complementary or differing perspectives.

▨ Consent forms contain a description of the research study and information about risks, the voluntary nature of the study, and the confidentiality of patient information. They specify benefits of participating and contact information for an independent institutional representative whom the study participant can get in touch with if necessary.

DISCUSSION QUESTIONS AND ACTIVITIES

1. Define *quantitative research*. Provide an example of quantitative research and draw a graph or a picture or in other ways illustrate what quantitative research means to you.

2. Conduct a literature review to identify an instrument that has been validated. What is the underlying construct that is being measured? What do the authors describe as the process for determining reliability? What reliability is reported?

3. Name and describe the population characteristics that would influence your choice of methods when conducting an evaluation of a recently instituted advocacy process to increase access to dental care for children of low-income families.

4. You are asked to assess the changes that occur following an initiative in your community. Describe the methods you would use and the approaches you would take to ensure a valid and reliable process for data collection and interpreting the data.

5. Identify a theme of your choice. What variables would fully describe the theme? Identify three of the most important indicators for measuring the theme, and write three to five questions for each theme. Develop your questions into a formatted questionnaire. Administer the questionnaire to a few of your friends or colleagues. Ask them to provide feedback on content, flow, and understanding. What important lessons did you learn from this process?

KEY TERMS

consent form
Institutional Review Board
interval-level data
nominal-level data
ordinal-level data
pilot testing
population sampling
qualitative data

qualitative research
quantitative data
quantitative research
ratio-level data
reliability
surveys
triangulation
validity

ANALYZING AND INTERPRETING THE DATA

QUANTITATIVE

LEARNING OBJECTIVES

- Analyze quantitative data.
- Interpret quantitative data and reach conclusions.

Quantitative data analysis is the systematic examining of the evidence that is collected in answering a specific research question. It is the process of sorting and categorizing data using the appropriate tools and approaches. The third step of the Participatory Model for Evaluation is to analyze and interpret the data (Figure 8.1). This chapter discusses how quantitative data are analyzed and interpreted to answer the evaluation question.

Interpreting the data to reach appropriate, defensible, and sound conclusions about the evaluation requires that the evaluation be supported by good-quality data and suitable analyses. It means making judgments about the initiative's merits, value, or worth to the program beneficiaries, the program staff, the community, and the funders. Reaching conclusions results in recommendations for decision making about the initiative.

ANALYZING AND REPORTING QUANTITATIVE DATA

The type of data collected during a research study determines the type of analysis that can be undertaken. The data collected in survey research is most often categorized as categorical, dichotomous, or continuous. Nominal variables constitute categorical data, while dichotomous data indicate the absence or presence of the characteristic being measured. Examples of pairs of dichotomous variables are healthy/not healthy, well/not well (sick), male/not male (female). In this case, "healthy" may be coded as 1 for data entry, while "not healthy" is coded as 2. Dichotomous variables like nominal-scale data have limited options in data analysis.

FIGURE 8.1.   *The Participatory Framework for Evaluation: Analyze and Interpret the Data*

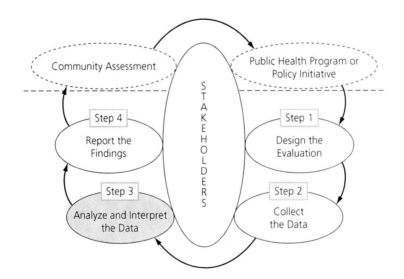

Ordinal variables that are used in ranking the indicator provide for more sophisticated analysis than do nominal-scale categorical variables. Continuous data allow for more detailed analysis than either nominal or ordinal data. If required, the flexibility of continuous data allows data to be grouped to produce categories and treated as ordinal data for analysis. For example, twenty children whose heights range from forty-eight inches to sixty-eight inches can be grouped into two categories. The first group would be children forty-eight inches to fifty-eight inches, and the second group would be children fifty-nine inches to sixty-eight inches.

Quantitative data can be analyzed in two ways—as descriptive statistics and as inferential statistics. The initial analysis in a research study produces descriptive statistics, which summarize and describe the data. These measures include:

- Frequencies, percentages, and proportions

- Measures of central tendency (mean, mode, and median)

- Measures of dispersion (range, standard deviations, variance)

Frequencies represent the number of times an event occurs or the number of responses, while percentages represent the number of occurrences or the number of responses as a proportion of the whole. For example, if thirty people respond to a survey out of a total of one hundred, the frequency of respondents is thirty, the proportion is 0.3, and the percentage is 30 percent. Each question in the survey, however, may have a different denominator for calculating percentages if all the questions are not answered. If, for example, question 20 was answered by only sixty people, then the denominator for calculating the proportion and hence the percentage is sixty.

Means are the most often used measure of central tendency. The mean is the calculated average of the responses. For example, if thirty people have scores ranging from ten to thirty, all the scores are totaled and the total is divided by thirty to calculate the mean. Means are also used to summarize the responses on rating scales. Modes are the most frequently occurring response, and medians are the middle value of a set of values with an equal number of values falling above and below.

The range is the span between the lowest and the highest scores. Standard deviations represent the variations in the data and the distance that the data points are from the mean. A low standard deviation indicates little difference between the value and the means of all the values, and a high standard deviation indicates a large difference. When there is no difference, the standard deviation is zero. Variance is the square of the standard deviation.

The first step in data analysis is to summarize the data across all the demographic variables and the survey items. In this first step, calculate frequencies, percentages, measures of central tendency, and measures of dispersion. Data analysis can be conducted in the data-analysis software Microsoft Excel® or SPSS® or other suitable computer software. The greater the variability in the data the more likely it is that the data can be explained and conclusions can be drawn about the relationship among the variables and about the population as a whole. The statistics calculated will be determined by the type of data you are working with. For example, you could do a mean for age because ages are continuous data, but a mean for gender, which is categorical, would be meaningless. For gender you would be limited to frequency and percentages, so look at the proportion of men compared with the proportion of women in the sample.

The results of the analysis can be presented in a variety of ways, including tables, charts, and graphs. In reporting the data, it is not sufficient to use graphics alone; they must be accompanied by narratives explaining what they mean to the reader. Providing the charts allows readers to also make their own interpretations of the data.

The following four examples illustrate ways of presenting and explaining data.

Example 1. Data presented in a table format (Table 8.1)

Analysis: There were a total of fifty-one participants in the study, most of whom (75 percent) were male.

Example 2. Data presented in a single-table format summarizing all the categories in the data (Table 8.2)

Analysis: A total of 160 men aged thirty-one to seventy-one (mean 56.7 years) were included in this study. Most of them (60 percent) were white, 25 percent were African American, and 15 percent were Hispanic of Mexican origin. Most (95 percent) were satisfied with the program, with a mean satisfaction score of 4.69 on a five-point scale, and 94 percent said they would recommend the program to somebody else.

Example 3. Data presented in a bar-chart format (Figure 8.2)

Analysis: Overall, participants were satisfied with all the activities. Mean score for the physical-activity component was 4.5; for nutrition education it was slightly less at 4.0; and participants walking with their peers it was 3.6. Although there was no significant difference in satisfaction scores between the nutrition activity and the in-gym activities, there was a significant difference between the in-gym activities and the participants walking with their peers ($p = .02$).

Example 4. Data presented in a pie-chart format (Figure 8.3)

Analysis: There were almost equal numbers of participants in the three offerings of the initiatives.

Cross-tabulations are a useful way to summarize data in bivariate relationships. They can be used with nominal or ordinal data. When used with nominal data, the statistic associated with them is the chi square, and when used with ordinal data, the statistic is known as Spearman's Rank Order Correlation.

Analyzing data from quasi-experiments consists primarily of comparing the intervention group with the comparison group against the outcome variable. Inferential statistics describe the analysis that makes inferences about the data and a population from

TABLE 8.1. **Single-Variable Table Format for Presenting Quantitative Data**

Response Category	Frequency (*N*)	Percentage (%)
Male	38	74.5
Female	13	25.5
Total	51	100

TABLE 8.2. **Multiple-Variable Table Format for Presenting Quantitative Data**

Sample Characteristic	Response Category	Number of Participants *N* = 160	Percentage (%)
Age (years)	Sample mean = 56.7		
Race/Ethnicity	AA/Black	41	26
	Hispanic	24	15
	White	95	59
Satisfaction with the program	Yes	152	95
	No	8	5
Satisfaction with program	Mean score = 4.69		
1 = Not at all satisfied	1	3	2
2 = Somewhat dissatisfied	2	5	3
3 = Neutral	3	0	0
4 = Somewhat satisfied	4	60	38
5 = Very Satisfied	5	92	57
Recommendation to others	Yes	150	94
	No	2	1
	Maybe	8	5

FIGURE 8.2. *Bar-Chart Format for Presenting Quantitative Data*

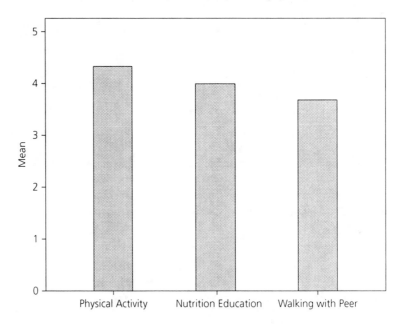

FIGURE 8.3. *Pie-Chart Format for Presenting Quantitative Data*

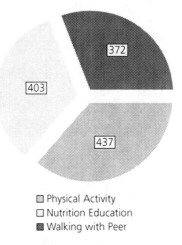

☐ Physical Activity
☐ Nutrition Education
▨ Walking with Peer

the sample that is studied. Estimation and hypothesis testing are inferential statistics where the null hypothesis determines whether there is a true difference between the two groups being compared (Jekel, Elmore, & Katz, 1996). If the participants in the sample were not randomly assigned and the assumption cannot be made that the results are generalizable to a larger population, inferential statistics may be inappropriate.

A commonly used test to assess the difference in means before and after evaluation designs is the paired t-test. The z-test is used to compare differences between proportions in a group that has received an intervention compared with a group that did not. A fuller description of these and other statistical tests that may be used in evaluation include the chi-square test, ANOVA, and bivariate and multivariate analysis are beyond the scope of this book.

REACHING CONCLUSIONS

Because evaluation is primarily about assessing the initiative's merit, worth, or value, the analysis of the data is used to formulate the conclusion. Conclusions are based on criteria developed at the start of the process and on the standards that were established by the evaluation team and the stakeholders. The synthesis of the results of an evaluation study requires the integration of all the results that are obtained from the many assessments that may have been carried out. In addition to the data being interpreted to reflect statistical significance, the data must also be interpreted to reflect practical significance and importance to the stakeholders in the light of their values and standards. Developing a summary of the data and the analysis will help in organizing and synthesizing the information.

The aim is to present a balanced report that discusses the value of the initiative to the different stakeholder audiences. The value of the initiative may be both tangible and intangible and is assessed using multiple criteria that include:

- Relevant information about the initiative (description and context)

- Objective, unbiased, and systematic research

- Performance on indicators of merit in process and outcome measures

- Recognized standards and criteria of performance based on comparison groups or other programs or both

- Cost-efficiency criteria

- Policies, regulations, and laws

- Stakeholder and community values and expectations

- Environmental standards

- Standards of social justice and equity

In addition to being assessed against expected outcomes, the data are also assessed for unexpected outcomes that benefit or hurt the community, participants, or nonparticipants.

Lessons learned from conducing the evaluation are identified. They pertain to the value of the evaluation, the range of experiences in the research approach, participant recruitment, data collection, and research findings. Assessing failures or shortcomings of the evaluation provides an opportunity to plan improvements in the evaluation process.

STAKEHOLDER INVOLVEMENT

Members of the community are much less likely to want to be involved in data analysis than in the data-collection phase of the evaluation. However, they can play a number of roles, and their contributions need not be any less than in any other phase of the evaluation. In the spirit of Community-Based Participatory Research and empowerment, it is important that data-analysis skills be taught. The team may need to bring in new members from the community who are both interested in and have the aptitude to learn the methods; quantitative-data analysis requires background knowledge that usually comes with a higher level of academic preparation.

STEPS IN QUANTITATIVE-DATA ANALYSIS AND INTERPRETATION

Let us review a process for thinking about an evaluation research study. The evaluator was part of the process from the very beginning and wanted to be sure the group started out knowing as much as they could about the group before designing an intervention.

Background: The rates of transmission of sexually transmitted diseases were increasing again after a few years of a slow decline in spite of the fact that a range of educational programs were being offered. In preparation for another intervention, it was decided to conduct an assessment of the most vulnerable population, the population where the rates of infection appear to be increasing the most. The assessment was designed to provide information on which to base the intervention. The population of interest was a youthful, computer-savvy group that used social networking extensively. Because the intervention was to be implemented through a social-networking mechanism, the computer-based assessment was conducted using the same site. The assumption was that the group that got the survey would be fairly representative of the group that would get the intervention.

Methodology: The researchers designed a survey that consisted of a number of sections. They collected demographic data, including age, ethnicity, gender, marital status, state and county of residence, alcohol and other drug use, sexual preferences, sexual risk behaviors, and knowledge and attitudes about practices related to the transmission and prevention of sexually transmitted diseases. In addition they asked questions about the practicality of using social-networking sites to conduct an intervention.

The evaluators distributed the previously validated IRB approved survey with a cover letter explaining the intent of the study and provided a link that respondents could click on if they were interested. Within the next few days they received eighteen hundred responses.

Data analysis: The survey generated a combination of categorical and continuous data that were downloaded, transferred into SPSS®, and checked for entry errors. Discrepancies were resolved, and the data were cleaned. The evaluation team calculated frequencies on all categorical variables and the means on all appropriate categories. The chi square was used to test associations of categorical variables. The alpha level for statistical significance was set to 0.05. The evaluators were interested in knowing whether the subgroups within the sample differed in any meaningful way, so they created subsamples and compared them using ANOVA.

Describing the data: The data analysis allowed a description of the sample including a demographic profile and knowledge, attitudes, and practices regarding the transmission and prevention of sexually transmitted diseases. In addition, risk and protective factors were identified as well as social and political determinants of health. Tables and charts were created to show the characteristics of the respondents and the results of the tests that were run with their corresponding *p*-values.

The results provided researchers with information about the specific characteristics of subgroups within the sample, and significant differences were detected. The eighteen- to twenty-four-year-olds were significantly different in their risk-taking behaviors from the groups that were twenty-five to thirty and thirty-one to thirty-five. In addition, the level of risk-taking behaviors was associated with alcohol consumption, and there was a difference in the type of risk taking by group and the behaviors that they engaged in.

Interpreting the data: The group with fairly high risk-taking behavior was college students. Overall, they were less inclined toward prevention of sexually transmitted disease and more likely to consume alcohol than those in the older groups. They were much more likely to believe that a cure was available for each of the sexually transmitted diseases and less likely to believe they were at risk for infection from their practices.

Following a full review of the results, the team decided to design different interventions for each age group. Even though the eighteen- to twenty-four-year olds presented the greatest risk, the thirty-one to thirty-five-year olds exhibited risk behaviors that were different but also had to be addressed. Because the largest group that participated in the study was the college-age group, the team concluded that the first intervention designed would be for them. This intervention would serve as a pilot.

The team compared their findings with those of other researchers. They reviewed the literature again to be sure they had not missed any recent papers and found that although their study had been conducted online, their results were not significantly different from the results of studies that had been conducted on college campuses. They found it surprising that, unlike previous studies, their study showed no differences among the three ethnic groups that dominated the sample. This was an especially important finding for the researchers and planners because their intervention would be online and they would have much less control over who would take part. They decided to institute a password-secured site for the intervention. They knew that young people shared a lot of information with their friends, including passwords to online programs, so controlling access would be challenging. The team used results about the social, cultural, and political context to guide the development of the intervention and to decide how they would implement and evaluate their work over a three-year funding period.

SUMMARY

- Descriptive statistics summarize and describe the data. Frequencies, percentages, measures of central tendency (mean, median, mode), and measures of dispersion (standard deviations, variance) are used for descriptive analyses.

- The method of analysis is determined by the characteristics of the data and the combination of levels of measurement across the outcome and the intervention variable. The most commonly used analysis for comparing two groups is the mean.

- Data must be interpreted based on criteria developed at the start of the process and on the standards that were established by the evaluation team and the stakeholders.

- The data must also be interpreted to reflect their practical significance and importance to the stakeholders in light of their values and standards.

DISCUSSION QUESTIONS AND ACTIVITIES

1. Identify a small data set. Summarize the data manually or using a data-analysis software package. Write a short report describing the data in terms of each of the variables. What analyses did you use? What conclusions did you draw from your findings?

2. Conduct a literature review and find two research articles. Read the articles and write a short summary describing the variables in the data and the analyses that were conducted. How were the results of the analysis displayed? What conclusions did the authors draw from their results?

 ## KEY TERMS

descriptive statistics	measures of dispersion
frequencies	mode
mean	standard deviation
measures of central tendency	variance

COLLECTING THE DATA

QUALITATIVE

LEARNING OBJECTIVES

- Describe data collection in qualitative research.
- Describe reliability and validity in qualitative research.

Qualitative-research methods can be used in program evaluation as the precursor to the development of a survey, to understand the extent to which programs are implemented, or to determine whether the intervention activities caused a change in program participants. They can be used to understand the context of the initiative and to identify the theory on which the program was developed. Qualitative-research approaches increase the participation of those who are less powerful in the community and give them a voice.

Qualitative research relies on one or a combination of approaches and tools. The selection of the approach or the tool depends on the type of study, what you need to know, and often on the perspective or the training and orientation of the researcher. Creswell (2007, p. 1) describes how a project changed considerably with the input of an ethnographic perspective from a cultural anthropologist.

In public health program evaluation, although all qualitative-research approaches are used to a greater or lesser degree, the tools that have largely been adopted are case studies, focus-group discussions, individual interviews, participant and nonparticipant observation (drawing on the art and science of ethnography), and record reviews. Community-Based Participatory Research methods such as photovoice and digital storytelling have been adopted as well. This chapter reviews qualitative approaches with interview, document-review, observational, case-review, digital, and Geographic Information System formats.

QUALITATIVE DATA

The primary value of using qualitative data-collection approaches rather than quantitative data-collection approaches in evaluation is the difference in the role the interviewer plays in soliciting information when interviewing techniques are used. In quantitative interviewing, the interview is strictly scripted and consists primarily of closed-ended questions. In qualitative-data collection, interviewers ask open-ended questions that allow for elaboration of the responses and require the interviewer to master the skills of asking questions, listening carefully, and interpreting the responses to the questions. Conducting qualitative research also requires the development of a protocol. Protocols ensure consistency across the interviews, which increases the reliability of the findings. The protocol contains the following items:

- The interviewer's opening remarks

- The process for getting informed consent

- The process for conducting the interview

- The process for completing paperwork related to the interview. including a time sheet, perceptions of the interaction and the degree of reliability of the respondent, and the data

The main disadvantage of qualitative data is in the small sample size; in addition, for the analysis large volumes of interview data have to be transcribed and coded for themes and patterns.

Giacomini and Cook (2000) identify the essential aspects of qualitative research as appropriate participant selection and comprehensive, appropriate data collection that is corroborated by multiple sources.

ENSURING VALIDITY AND RELIABILITY

An important consideration in the collection of qualitative data is its validity and reliability. Alternative terms are that the data be *trustworthy* and *dependable* (Ulin, Robinson, & Tolley, 2005). Validity is equated with credibility and with the extent to which the approach is appropriate for answering the research question (Fern, 2001) and the extent to which the data measure the concepts that they are intended to measure. It assumes that the concepts are appropriately defined based on an accurate understanding of the context and that the findings and conclusions are consistent with the data that are collected and are believable by the stakeholders, who consider them to be accurate (Ulin et al., 2005, p. 25). Conclusions drawn from the data may be invalid if there is bias in the theoretical frameworks, the preconceptions of the researcher, or in the selection of particular parts of the data for emphasis when the results are compiled. An important aspect of evaluation that allows for diverse and culturally appropriate interpretations and increased validity is the emphasis on stakeholder involvement in the entire process (Nelson-Barber, LeFrance, Trumbull, & Aburto, 2005). Additional considerations for increasing validity include:

- Collecting data rich enough to provide a complete picture

- Soliciting feedback from the respondents about the data and the conclusions that are drawn from the data

- Searching for discrepant evidence and negative cases in the data to reduce selection bias

- Triangulating data sources, settings, and methods thus reducing the chance of a systematic bias in the method and assuring the generalizability of the conclusions

- Comparing intervention and comparison/control groups in a quasi-experimental/experimental design across different settings (Maxwell, 2005)

Reliability in qualitative research is associated with dependability and the extent to which the data-collection approaches are thorough and follow recognized rules and conventions. Questions associated with reliability include:

- Are the research purpose and design logically connected to the data gathered?

- Are the results complemented by data from other sources?

- Are the interviews conducted by trained interviewers using uniform approaches specified by protocols? (Ulin et al., 2005)

If data are dependable, the relationship between the data and the findings across multiple methods and over time will remain stable. Qualitative research requires that the researcher remain objective and report any conflict of values to the evaluation team because they may influence the collection, analysis, and interpretation of the data resulting in a bias.

INTERVIEW-FORMAT APPROACHES

Focus-Group Discussions

A focus group is a moderated group interaction used to conduct research that relies on the interaction of participants in the group to produce the data. Focus groups are used for a variety of reasons that include:

- Deepening understanding of a phenomenon or a community

- Gathering information about the range of knowledge, opinions, experiences, attitudes, and beliefs of a group

- Understanding broad themes

Focus-group interviews can be used at each stage of the evaluation. The focus-group interview is a structured process conducted by a trained facilitator who utilizes open-ended questions to solicit information in a face-to-face format. Participants in a focus group inform the research and provide data on topics of which they have a personal or professional understanding. Telephone and computer-facilitated focus groups have been used by academic researchers to reach dispersed population groups and to provide anonymity to the respondents (Abbatangelo-Gray, Cole, & Kennedy, 2007; Cooper, Jorgensen, & Meritt, 2003).

Six to eight individuals form a purposefully selected group to participate in a focus-group discussion. The specific purposes are to gather information, uncover perspectives, and elicit the factors that influence opinions, motivations, or behavior (Krueger & Casey, 2000). In some research and across world cultures, gender or other homogeneity in the group is critically important to consider. Fern (2001) suggests that homogeneity is probably more important with regard to socioeconomic status than it is to race/ethnicity. In some instances a heterogeneous group may be appropriate, depending on the research questions. Discussion within the group provides the intergroup checking of information, increasing the validity of the data.

Like other research methodologies, focus groups have unique characteristics.

- They provide rich qualitative data.

- They can be used to understand a phenomenon of interest more fully than survey techniques.

- Direct quotations from the interview provide powerful imagery for the reader when focus-group data are reported.

Limitations in using focus groups for evaluation research must also be considered.

- Focus groups are small groups of six to eight people who may not be representative of the larger population, and results may not be generalizable beyond the sample. Probability sampling from a stratified sample will increase the generalizability of the sample if the final sample is sufficiently heterogeneous even while maintaining in-group homogeneity (Fern, 2001).

- It can be difficult and time consuming to assemble focus groups.

- Focus groups require respondents to commit to spending one to two hours in the interview.

- Focus groups are unsuitable for collecting sensitive information or in situations where the topic is emotionally charged or likely to lead to contention.

Other potentially important drawbacks of the focus-group method include the strong possibility that the moderator will bias the discussion and the difficulty of separating individual viewpoints from the collective group viewpoint. In a focus group, individuals may be less willing to reveal sensitive information because assurance of confidentiality is lost when participants may know each other from work or other social contexts. Providing opportunities for social integration before the group discussion increases the level of comfort group members have with each other (Fern, 2001). An ice-breaker at the start of this interview may also serve this purpose.

The Facilitator   The role of focus-group facilitators is to moderate, not to dominate or to participate in, the discussion. Their role is to ask the questions and to be sure that everybody participates. It is important that the group discussion not be dominated by any one individual. Not allowing one or two persons to dominate the discussion requires skill and patience.

The facilitator may take notes, but having a note taker allows the facilitator to focus on moderating the discussion. The note taker not only records statements made by participants but may also keep track of the participants' choice of words, nonverbal communications, expressions of emotion, and the roles played by participants.

When conducting a number of focus groups, it is important to use the same facilitator or to ensure training of all the facilitators in order to control for the influence of the facilitator and to improve the reliability of the data.

Conducting a Focus-Group Discussion   The interview starts with an opening question that serves as an icebreaker. It can be as simple as, "Tell me what it is like to live in this neighborhood." The rest of the interview consists of eight to ten open-ended questions built around a particular theme and developed to answer the research question. It may consist of probes that allow for an increased understanding of the phenomenon being studied and provides prompts for the researcher. A probe for the previous example could be, How is it similar to or different from previous neighborhoods you have lived in? Additional probes to get at what participants are thinking or to expand the discussion include, Would you explain that further?, Would you say more about that?, Tell me more about that.

The following steps are involved in conducting a focus group:

- Confirm the purpose of the study and the problem it is addressing.

- Ensure the individual questions are conversational, short, and clear and contain only one dimension. Use probes to expand the options for questioning.

- Organize the logistics, including establishing the interview time line, securing a venue, purchasing recording equipment and supplies, arranging for participant or community incentives, developing advertising flyers if appropriate.

- Recruit and train the facilitator and note taker.

- Contact and recruit the potential study population by appropriate methods including letters, e-mails, flyers placed in appropriate venues, phone calls.

- Confirm the time and location.

- Convene the group and ensure that each person provides informed consent to participate and for the interview to be recorded.

- Conduct the focus-group interview.

- Close the interview.

Detailed guidance for conducting focus groups is provided in Krueger and Casey (2000).

Individual Interviews

Individual interviews are used to get information about an individual's participation in or exposure to a public health program or about the impact of a policy or about attitudes, feelings, and behaviors related to a public health problem. Key informants provide insights about a situation or a population from their own vantage point. They may also provide information about resources and services. They are often community leaders such as heads of agencies, heads of institutions, policymakers, and service providers. Key informants often have a perspective that is different from the perspectives of program participants.

When a member of the community or a program participant is less likely to be invited to participate in a focus group of peers because he or she holds strong views or is likely to polarize the group, an individual interview is a great alternative. Unlike questionnaire administration, individual interviews require a considerable amount of human capital for data collection; they are time consuming and expensive.

Advantages and Disadvantages   There are advantages and disadvantages to using individual interviews. Benefits include:

- The interviewer is able to ask additional questions, called *probes*, to improve a response or to ask for clarification of an answer.

- Interviewers can elicit sensitive information.

- The views and opinions of nonreaders and those with low literacy levels are easily incorporated into the study.

  Limitations include:

- Individual interviews are expensive because of the need to hire interviewers, provide travel expenses, and compensate respondents for their time.

- Scheduling interviews may be difficult, and potential respondents may not be easily recruited.

- The number of interviews may be small, although data may provide a considerable amount of depth and understanding. A small sample size makes it difficult to extrapolate the findings much beyond the sampled population.

- Rapport between the interviewer and the person being interviewed must be achieved before an interview because it affects the quality of the data.

Conducting an Individual Interview   Individual interviews can be carried out face-to-face at a time and in a place agreed to by both the interviewer and the respondent; the need for both privacy and safety should be taken into account. Individual interviews are held in neutral locations such as a local library, community center, or any space that is comfortable and that the participant perceives as nonthreatening; private and safe locations allow discussions of especially sensitive topics in an atmosphere of anonymity and confidentiality. Interviews may be conducted in the interviewee's home or office. Conducting a telephone interview eliminates some of the costs in time and travel but has limitations in building rapport with the respondent.

Recording an in-person or a telephone interview minimizes the risk of missing important information and distracting the respondent by writing extensive notes. Good digital recorders provide excellent recording quality. The interviewer seeks permission to record the interview during the initial discussions and makes this permission part of the informed-consent process. Permission is usually granted if a clear explanation is given such as, "It is important that this interview be recorded so I can listen to you and not be distracted by taking notes, and also to be sure I don't miss anything you say." Videotaping has become popular with qualitative researchers. Although members of some communities may not object to having an audio interview, many will not agree to be videotaped for fear of how the video images may be used in the future. Previous experiences or skepticism about the research method may influence their concerns.

Irrespective of the approach, conducting a good interview takes preparation. Individual interviews require the interviewer to be a skilled listener and communicator and a good researcher.

Designing the Interview Instrument Designing the instrument for an individual interview starts with having a clearly defined purpose and research question: What is it that you want to know? Once the research question is defined, the next task is to define the concepts and indicators that are related to the question. The third step in this process is to frame the specific questions that will be asked.

To give an example: The research question is, "Did the initiatives to improve access to care make a difference for the residents?" The initiatives are to improve access to care through two approaches. One, a provision in an existing policy, would allow more people to be eligible for health care based on poverty guidelines, and the other is a new primary health care facility within ten miles of 50 percent of the community's residents. Indicators for answering the evaluation question include knowledge of the policy, registrations under the policy, opinions about and use of the new health care facility, and the receipt of services. Alternatively, the questions that need to be answered may be about the theory-based intervention that was undertaken. In this case, the questioning in the evaluation is guided by the changes that were anticipated based on the Theory of Change. In the example of access to care, using qualitative research approaches could lead to questions such as:

▨   What do you know about the recent changes in the policy to increase eligibility?

▨   How do you believe the changes in the policy affect utilization of health care by residents of your county?

▨   What do you know about the clinic that was opened in your community recently?

▨   What is your opinion of the clinic?

▨   How has the clinic changed the lives of residents of this community?

▨   How have clinic usage patterns changed since the institution of the new policy?

An alternative approach to asking questions is using a short vignette to present a problem to which the interviewee or participants in the focus group can respond. The question, "What do you know about the clinic that was opened in your community recently?" is converted to a vignette format and becomes, " There have been many different reactions, both positive and negative, to the recently opened clinic in your community. What do you know about the clinic and its services and how did it affect access to health care in this community?"

Questions must be clear, must reflect the concept being measured accurately, and must be appropriately worded to elicit both depth and breadth in the responses. They must be asked in a logical sequence to allow the respondent to build on a train of thought and go from broad to specific questions. The time taken to develop a well-designed instrument for individual interviews or focus-group discussions is time well spent.

Sample Size

The number of focus groups and individual interviews that are conducted may be prescribed by the research questions and the number of groups and individuals across whom the data are to be compared. It may also depend on the likelihood that each successive group or interview will provide the same information. Once the same information is being gathered, *saturation* is reached, and the data collection may end (Krueger & Casey, 2000).

A study of "attitudes toward health care utilization" will require more groups or individuals to get at all the phenomena and the variability across subgroups than a research question on "adolescent girls' preferences for exercise," for instance. The first question is much broader and covers a wide range of individuals who may have differing attitudes toward health care utilization either as consumers or as service providers. The second research question, on adolescent girls, is more focused and conceivably has less variability; therefore saturation is likely to be reached sooner. Although interviews are generally conducted only once with any one group or individual during a single research study, the same group or individual may be interviewed in follow-up conversations if the phenomena or situation changes or in the conduct of case studies.

Appreciative Inquiry

Appreciative Inquiry is a specific use of interviewing skills in evaluation. It is defined as "a group of processes that inquires into, identifies, and further develops the best of 'what is' in organizations in order to create a better future" (Preskill & Catsambas, 2006, p. 1). Appreciative Inquiry is implemented in four phases: inquire, imagine, innovate, and implement. The inquire and imagine phases are most applicable to the data-collection phase of evaluation. An individual, paired, or group interview technique is used with a storytelling approach to obtain the following information:

- Experiences that most represent a participant's pride in being part of the initiative

- What participants value most about themselves and the program, processes, and successes

- Three things participants especially wish for the program

- Recommendations for improving outcomes

In the inquire phase, respondents are asked specifically to think back on their experience and tell a story. Preskill and Catsambas (2006, p. 80) give an example:

> *Think back on your experience in the workshop and tell me about a moment when you felt that a program or activity was working particularly well, so well that it helped you learn and understand the content in a way that was exciting or inspiring. What was it that made it so effective? What value did you add to the workshop? If the entire workshop were designed to be this clear, interesting, and engaging, what three wishes would you offer the workshop's designers to make this possible?*

The stories obtained during this process define success: how well the organization's systems work and how participants experience the initiative. The stories allow for a shared understanding and clarification of the program's culture.

The imagine phase encourages participants to provide information that helps frame the recommendations. The innovate phase produces concrete steps for improving the initiative and shaping systems and relationships differently. The innovate phase moves the initiative toward making changes if necessary. Given the wide range of questions in this approach, it may be used to answer process as well as outcome evaluation questions.

DOCUMENT AND RECORD REVIEW

Document and record review is especially important in process evaluation, when the evaluation questions focus on whether the initiative was implemented as planned and who the participants were. It may also be important in outcome evaluation. In the assessment of medical services, for example, medical records may be reviewed to understand the extent of family-support services. Case reviews may be conducted to assess the use of referrals and the utilization of services.

Documents reviewed for assessing program implementation can include:

- The plan for the initiative to determine the extent to which the plan was implemented as stated

- Existing needs-assessment data and reports to understand the sociocultural, economic, and epidemiological foundations of the program

- Minutes of board, executive committee, and ad hoc committee meetings to understand various aspects of program implementation and actions taken as well as ad hoc reports that may have been produced

- Meeting and training logs of participation in the initiative

- Logs of program implementation and any changes in implementation that occurred over time

- Photographs and videos that provide evidence of decisions made, actions taken, and level of participation

▓ Training curricula, teaching and learning resources for training program beneficiaries and providers

OBSERVATIONAL APPROACHES

Observation as a complement to qualitative or quantitative research approaches is an
important tool for evaluation. Observations may be made about behaviors, relationships, physical structures, conditions, sociocultural activities, and events. Ulin et al.
(2005, p. 72) comment that "observation is the oldest and most basic source of human
knowledge, from causal understanding of the everyday world to its use as a systematic
tool of social science." Observations are conducted using two approaches, the observer
as "insider" and the observer as "outsider." The more often used approach in evaluation is the unobtrusive observer as outsider.

This approach is used to understand or determine an outcome through observing
its occurrence (Ulin et al., 2005); alternatively it may be used to assess the implementation of an initiative and provide information during process or outcome evaluation.
In answering the research question, Did the initiatives improve access to care for residents?, the evaluators may choose to observe particular utilization events, such as the
reception and treatment of a subgroup of the population that usually experiences dis-
crimination when requiring care. Evaluators may observe

▓ patients from their entry into the facility to when they leave, taking note of multiple interactions with all levels of personnel

▓ the length of time patients are in the waiting room as well as in other parts of the
clinic

▓ the availability of culturally and developmentally appropriate reading materials,
videos, and other types of information sharing

▓ the number, types, and accessibility of other similar facilities within the
community

Data quality is improved by developing a carefully validated checklist with appropriate categories and by carefully observing the phenomena under study. The longer
the period of observation, the more credible the data because people will eventually
return to their natural behaviors. Data may be collected using checklists with space for
short comments; the checklists can be on small cards (Ulin et al., 2005) or in a
notebook.

The development of an observational checklist should include the participation of
stakeholders who have the ability to provide unique perspectives on the community
and to understand the meaning and relevance of behaviors and conditions for health
(Zenk, Schulz, House, Benjamin, & Kannan, 2005). Walking tours to understand
issues related to improvements for pedestrians using walkability-assessment tools provide an excellent combination of observation, surveys, and interviewing techniques.

Following each data-collection activity additional observations or interpretations can be added to the data. The data are analyzed to reflect both qualitative and quantitative dimensions as appropriate.

CASE REVIEWS

A case review describes the problem that is being addressed and discusses the activities that are being undertaken to address the problem. It is a focused, in-depth analysis of a program or system. The evaluation looks at the program's geographical location; its cultural, organizational, and historical contexts; and its implementation (Stufflebeam & Shinkfield, 2007). Its primary purpose is to describe a program in specific and illuminative terms. In addition, it makes recommendations for future actions. Case reviews can be used for evaluating initiatives and providing a complete understanding of what happened and why. It focuses on the question, What is the program and how does it work? Because an individual case review is not generalizable, a group of programs that address a similar problem may be used together to develop a theoretical framework for addressing a problem.

Sources of information for case reviews include agency reports, key-informant and focus-group data, observation, site visits, activity-monitoring reports and project documents. In addition case-review evaluation may include digital data-collection approaches such as photovoice and digital storytelling.

DIGITAL APPROACHES

Photographic approaches to data collection add an additional set of tools to the evaluator's tool kit. Alternative approaches to interviewing include using photographs and other artifacts to stimulate discussion and to create meaning about the issue. These techniques lend themselves to the active participation of multiple stakeholders (Bender & Harbour, 2001; Wang et al., 1996). Like other qualitative approaches, these methods allow the participation and input of less powerful members of the community.

One approach is to present one or more photographs or other visual aids (Bender & Harbour, 2001) to a group or individual and then facilitate a discussion of what the photograph or artifact means to the participant(s) using a series of reflective questions. The alternative photovoice technique (Wang et al., 1996) allows community members to be active participants in documenting their observations; in using photography to elicit emotions, feelings, and insight; and in sharing their worldviews. Cameras are given to participants so that they can present their community and environment in visual form and discuss their findings in their own words. Using this approach stimulates discussion among multiple stakeholders and allows the evaluator to see the images through an alternate set of validating lenses.

Photographic approaches may be applied in outcome evaluation to demonstrate changes that occur over time in the community from initiatives that leave a visible impact and show distinct physical changes. Before- and- after photographs or video may be used to show changes in lighting to improve safety in a community or improvement in the structures in a park or on the roads to increase physical activity. Changes in conditions such as those that preserve or improve the social environment may also be presented.

Adapting these approaches to evaluation practice allows the evaluation team to

- identify and discuss the community's concerns before and after an initiative

- promote critical thinking about issues that are presented in the photographs or are represented by the artifacts

- understand the values associated with initiatives undertaken in the community

- discuss the results of an initiative in graphic terms to a mixed stakeholder audience

- triangulate data in assessing outcomes against the standards of the evaluation to improve the validity of the evaluation process

The systematic collection of data requires a set of defined actions that start with the research question and include describing the methodology, identifying the participants in the study, compiling the results of the data collection, and analyzing the data.

The S-H-O-W-E-D (Wallerstein & Burnstein, 1998) technique may be adapted to facilitate discussion in the evaluation of an initiative to address visible changes in a community by asking the following questions. (A more useful acronym in this adaptation would be S-H-E-D.)

What do you *see* in this photograph?

How do the conditions in this photograph relate to your lives?

How can we become more *empowered* by our new understanding?

What can we *do* to address these issues?

The responses to these questions may serve as a useful indication of the success or failure of the intervention. Furthermore, the participatory nature of this technique provides opportunities for discussion of continued action to improve conditions in addition to providing concrete and direct stakeholder input into the evaluation recommendations.

Digital storytelling has gained some recognition in evaluation and complements photovoice in data collection. It may be used to support the photography or may be used alone. In digital storytelling, stories of participants are recorded before and after an intervention or may be used during the community assessment phase of the evaluation process.

GEOGRAPHIC INFORMATION SYSTEMS

Geographic Information Systems (GIS) provide the ability to link foundation database information with health data for public health purposes. Readily available and widely used data sets include detailed street-level information as well as political and administrative information such as zip codes and census tracts. The layering of census data on public health data shows the relationship between socioeconomic factors and disease at the block or census level.

For example, a tuberculosis project showed the distribution of disease superimposed on high school completion rates and income levels, demonstrating that the distribution of tuberculosis is related to low high school graduation rates and low levels of income (Harris & López-Defede, 2004). This study combined interviewing, using a semi-structured format, and GIS mapping to understand the phenomena of interest.

TRAINING DATA COLLECTORS

Training is important for all qualitative methods to ensure validity and reliability in the data-collection approaches. Conducting qualitative interviews requires that moderators and facilitators be well trained and have an opportunity to practice interviewing and observation skills using the instrument. Training ensures that interviews move smoothly and that questions easily transition from one to the other. Training sessions are as long or as short as necessary and include:

- An introduction to the objectives of the evaluation

- A review of the data-collection techniques

- A review of the data-collection instruments

- Practice in using the interview or observation instrument(s)

- Practice of interviewing skills

- Logistics for the interview session, including mechanisms for obtaining consent, recording the session, and identifying participants during the session in the case of focus groups

In this participatory model of evaluation, community members of the team may be data collectors for the first time. In developing the content for the training, consideration must also be given to developing listening and summarizing skills. A needs assessment early in the process will provide information for the appropriate training content.

PILOT TESTING

Pilot testing a qualitative data collection instrument is a chance to determine whether and how it works under real-life conditions. It is a practice run for the real thing! It involves the interviewer or facilitator, a note taker if there is one, and respondents. Participants in the pilot test must be similar to the research-study participants.

Conducting the pilot test provides opportunities to test the flow of the questions and to familiarize the interviewer or focus-group facilitator with the research-study process and the questions. In addition, a pilot test may be used to ensure the validity of observation tools. It ensures that questions and observations are appropriate and culturally sensitive. In addition it allows recording equipment to be tested and the procedure to be timed.

Following the pilot test, the instrument is edited as necessary to change vocabulary, increase the sensitivity of the questions, and improve the flow. Once this process is complete, the instrument is ready to be used.

MANAGING AND STORING QUALITATIVE DATA

Audiotape or digital recordings from focus-group or individual interviews must be transcribed verbatim; notes taken of nonverbal communication during the interview may be written in to provide the context. Transcribing qualitative data is time consuming; if funding permits, this process can be contracted out to a transcription service. The transcription is reviewed by one or more members of the research team against the original recordings to add any words or statements that may have been missed in order to increase the credibility of the study.

If audio equipment is not used and the researcher relies on the interviewer or the facilitator and the note taker to compile the data, it is important that they do so as soon as possible after the data collection to ensure that as little information as possible is lost.

All data that are collected as part of the research study must be kept in a secure location accessible only to members of the evaluation team. Access may be restricted to those working directly on the data analysis. Signed consent forms and data must be kept separately, and no attempt can be made to link personal identifiers with the data in a study that promised anonymity and was approved by the Institutional Review Board under these conditions.

STAKEHOLDER INVOLVEMENT

The data-collection phase is traditionally the phase in which stakeholder involvement is most evident. In the Participatory Model for Evaluation, stakeholders are part of the process and are involved in tasks from identifying the research question to drawing conclusions about the findings. Stakeholders may be trained to collect all forms of qualitative data. Stakeholder involvement supports the selection of culturally appropriate data-collection approaches and the credibility of the findings.

SUMMARY

- Qualitative data collection may rely on one or a combination of approaches and tools. The selection of the approach or the tool depends on the type of study, on the type of information that needs to be collected, and, often, on the perspective and/or the training and orientation of the researcher.

- Qualitative-research tools that have largely been adopted are case studies, focus-group discussions, individual interviews, participant and nonparticipant observation drawing on the art and science of ethnography, and record reviews. Additional Community-Based Participatory Research methods include photovoice and digital storytelling.

- Validity and reliability are important in qualitative research. *Trustworthy* and *dependable* are terms used to describe validity; reliability is conceptualized as dependability and the extent to which the data are collected by using approaches that are thorough and follow recognized rules and conventions.

- Basic steps for conducting an interview are developing the instrument, organizing the logistics and training interviewers, piloting the instrument, contacting potential respondents, and conducting the interview.

DISCUSSION QUESTIONS AND ACTIVITIES

1. Define *qualitative research*. Provide an example of qualitative research and draw a graph, picture, or in other ways illustrate what qualitative research means to you.

2. Conduct a literature review to identify a qualitative-research study. What was being assessed? What was the process for conducting the research? How was validity assessed? What limitations of the study did the researchers identify?

3. Identify a research question of your choice. What qualitative approach(es) would you use to answer your research question? What assessment instruments would you develop? How would you ensure that your process is both valid and reliable?

KEY TERMS

focus group	qualitative research
individual interview	saturation
observation	stakeholders
photographic approaches	trustworthy
photovoice	validity

10

ANALYZING AND INTERPRETING THE DATA

QUALITATIVE

LEARNING OBJECTIVES

- Analyze different types of qualitative data.
- Interpret qualitative data and reach conclusions.

Qualitative-data analysis is the systematic examining of the evidence that is collected as a result of the research. It is the process of sorting and categorizing the data using the appropriate tools and approaches. Krueger and Casey (2000) define *focus-group analysis* as "systematic, verifiable, and continuous" (p. 128), and the same may be said about qualitative data that is produced in narrative form from individual interviews and through other forms of inquiry. The third step in the Participatory Model for Evaluation is analyzing and interpreting the data. This chapter discusses how qualitative data are analyzed and interpreted.

ANALYZING QUALITATIVE DATA

Text-Based Data

Qualitative research using interviewing approaches such as focus groups, individual interviews, appreciative inquiry, case studies, digital storytelling, or components of photovoice provides data that are converted into text through transcription. The next step in the process of handling this qualitative data is to reduce the quantity of information through a series of steps. Interview and focus-group instruments may provide the basis for the themes of the analysis, or themes may be identified in a grounded theory approach during the coding process. Analyzing the data provides the answers to the question(s) that generated the research and the data collection. The data may also be coded by categories such as time, event, person, place, thing. The data may be generated any number of ways to understand a phenomenon, a behavior, a service, an incident; but however it is generated the evaluator must identify and organize the information from the transcript or the text in a coherent manner.

Coding the data is done in multiple ways. One approach is to manually highlight the relevant or emerging themes in the category of interest in the printed document using a different color or pattern for each theme. The text that is highlighted in the same color may then be cut out and stacked to sort and organize the data, keeping the themes in designated piles. Throughout the process coding may lead to changes in the categories and renewed thinking about the analysis. It may sometimes lead to recoding all or parts of the transcript.

An alternative strategy is using computer-assisted data-coding and data-analysis software such as NVivo® or N6® from QSR, Ethnograph®, and ATLASti® (Figure 10.1). In addition, a cost-free resource, AnSWR (McLennan, Strotman, McGregor, & Dolan, 2004), is available at the CDC website: http://www.cdc.gov/hiv/topics/surveillance/resources/software/answr/index.htm. When computer-based software is used, themes are coded and text is linked to the data in much the same way as described above.

Four major advantages are associated with using a computer-based program:

1. The text that is coded stays linked to the main document.

2. The same segment of text may be coded for more than one theme.

3. The text can be easily recoded if necessary.

4. Intergroup analysis is facilitated because demographic attributes can be attached to the text.

FIGURE 10.1.   *Screen Shots of Qualitative-Data Coding from NVivo® QSR*

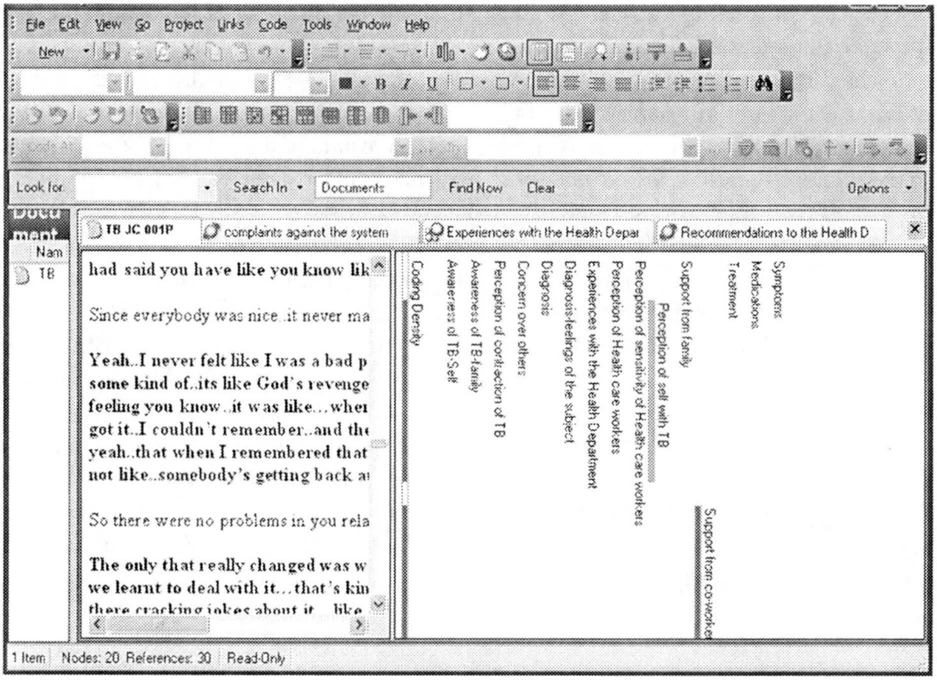

Coding and interpreting qualitative data is an iterative process that requires that the data be reviewed as it is being collected. It is important that the strategy for coding and analyzing the data be defensible and clearly documented.

In order to improve the reliability of the data-coding process, two to three people may be involved in the coding. Early in the process each person codes one to two interviews. The coders then come together to ensure that themes are being coded consistently and similarly based on a previously determined code/definitions protocol. The coders reconcile the codes, include new codes and definitions as needed, and decide on a single coding strategy that they all use for the rest of the transcribed interviews. Coders periodically review their work together until all the documents are coded. Alternative ways to sort and organize qualitative data are diagrams, charts, and graphs (Mason, 2002). A cognitive map that charts the data, much like the charting that can be achieved in computer-based coding, may be useful where interpretive themes are related to each other through tree, sister, and daughter codes, as in NVivo®.

Although determining the frequency of specific responses does not constitute an appropriate analysis of qualitative data, it is worth noting the number of people who mentioned the theme or the topic and the specificity with which different themes are discussed (Krueger & Casey, 2000). A more appropriate approach for quantifying qualitative data is to use phrases such as "some people," "most participants," "a few participants."

Once the coding process is complete, the themes are used to answer the evaluation research question and provide any additional insights that the data may reveal. This last step of interpreting the data requires explaining the meaning of the data, reporting the main ideas that the data reveal, and identifying important concepts.

The interpretations that are made and the conclusions that are drawn must reflect the data accurately to ensure credibility of the evaluation process. Responses to each question or emergent themes are compiled and the results of the study and the answers to the research questions are written up so readers can clearly see the data and be able to draw their own conclusions should they wish to do so.

Evaluators write up their reports by drawing on their knowledge of the data, their field notes, and their interpretation of the data through their own lenses. The write-up includes quotations that support the themes and the interpretation the evaluator is trying to convey. It is important to select quotations that illustrate a shared perception or opinion of the respondents. Select quotes from across the range of the data and use two to three to represent a theme (Krueger & Casey, 2000; Ulin et al., 2005). Quotations should represent the voices of participants. These quotes help readers feel close to the members of the community and increase their understanding of the experience. Quotations may also be used to highlight particular or interesting phenomena that may form the basis for further research but may not be typical of the views of most of the participants in the study.

EXAMPLE

USE OF QUOTES IN AN EVALUATION REPORT

In a qualitative study of the factors that influenced the treatment of tuberculosis, one of the themes identified was "social support during treatment." Part of the results section read as follows:

An important aspect of a treatment period is the support of family and friends. Participants in the study reported that they were well looked after while they were ill; some reported the tangible support of those who helped with household chores: *"My family . . . they were like pretty good. She [sister] stayed here with me. . . . She cooked for me."* Some individuals reported that friends and colleagues helped raise their spirits. One person said, *"The only thing that really changed was we started joking about it. . . . That was the way we learned to deal with it."*

Once the report is written, the researcher reconvenes the whole group and requests a review of the report, giving the evaluation team an opportunity to make any edits and ensure appropriate interpretation of the data. After this process is complete, the report may be made public.

Document and Record Reviews

The range of materials that may be included in document and record reviews allows for considerable flexibility in the selection of data-analysis tools. The analysis of medical records, minutes of meetings, or television commercials may necessitate the development of checklists on which the presence or absence of the phenomenon under study can be recorded.

Although this approach is primarily qualitative, it may also allow for the data to be categorized in diagrams, charts, and tables to allow for quantitative analysis, including determining means, frequencies, and so forth. In addition, the review can use quotes from participants or descriptions of the services provided. These data are handled in much the same way as text-based data, where themes are identified as the data are coded and interpreted.

Observational Methods

Observational methods may also utilize checklists or note-based formats with appropriate categories for recording events of interest. These data can be analyzed as quantitative data or can be used as descriptive data depending on the purpose of the study. A checklist may be combined with other qualitative research methods to provide evidence for making decisions.

In an observational approach to assess skill development based on a set of evaluative criteria, the observation tool lists the skill components, which can be rated on a five-point scale from poor performance of the skill to excellent performance of the skill. The data are analyzed as quantitative data, but in addition comments or individual interviews may be used to understand the participants' perceptions and intentions to use the skills following the training.

Geographic Information Systems Mapping

Multiple data sets may be used to analyze statistics and socioeconomic demographic data. Prevalence, incidence, and services data at county or zip code level can be used to analyze trends over time or to create a prevalence map. Socioeconomic variables may be used to determine both correlation and regression statistics for identifying the demographic groups that are most affected. Comparisons of health-related data and census data can be used to understand the extent of the problem. A team of student evaluators analyzed the data from eight counties served by a local nonprofit organization. By comparing their breast-cancer rates with state and national rates, the students were able to identify the counties with the greatest need for breast health services.

GIS mapping provides the opportunity to overlay data to understand interacting variables at multiple levels of analysis. It provides a pictorial perspective of data that are not otherwise available and demonstrates the relationships among variables of interest. The overlay of data may show the clustering of individuals with low socio-economic status based on low high school completion rates, low-paid jobs, female-headed households, and so forth. This information may provide an excellent complement to photographs and interviews reflecting the circumstances of disadvantaged communities.

INTERPRETING THE DATA AND REACHING CONCLUSIONS

Interpreting the data to reach conclusions allows the evaluation team to consider the following:

- The evidence for answering the evaluation question(s)

- The meaning of the results

- The practical significance of the results

When a combination of methods is used to answer a research question, the evaluator may have interview transcripts, photographs, digital recordings, and maps that represent different aspects of the data collection. All the data are organized to represent the theme or the question to facilitate interpretation.

Different stakeholder perspectives may influence the interpretation of qualitative data. These interpretations may be influenced by culture, age, demographics, life situation, or status as participants, staff, or funders. Funders, administrative staff, volunteers, and participants may look at the same quotations and draw different conclusions.

The aim is to present a balanced report of the conclusions that discusses the value of the initiative to the different stakeholder audiences. The value of the initiative may be both tangible and intangible and is assessed against any one or many of multiple criteria that include:

- Relevant information about the initiative (description and context)

- Objective, unbiased, and systematic research

- Performance on indicators of merit in process and outcome measures

- Recognized standards and criteria of performance based on comparison groups and/or other programs

- Cost and efficiency criteria

- Policies, regulations, and laws

- Stakeholder and community values and expectations

- Environmental standards

- Standards of social justice and equity

The compiled data are used to answer each research question in turn, using the objective that supports the research question as the standard for the final interpretation. For example, if the evaluation research question is, What factors influenced the reduced utilization of the emergency room for nonemergency health care and by how much was utilization reduced?, the supporting objective might read, One year after the clinic opening, utilization of the emergency room for nonemergency care will fall by 15 percent. Text-based data from individual interviews with members of the community, staff of the emergency room, and other key informants are used to understand the factors that influenced the reduced utilization of the emergency room, but complementary quantitative data are used to determine the level to which this reduction took place.

Conclusions about the value or worth of the intervention are based on the standard, in this case the objective(s). If the findings demonstrate that the initiative met or exceeded the standard(s), the initiative is said to be of value. In the example, the value may also be identified in cost-benefit terms to the emergency room as well as to the patients. If the objectives are not met, the conclusion might be that the initiative has little value and the investment was not worth the expenditure. The judgment is based entirely on the data that are collected, analyzed, and interpreted.

To illustrate how decisions about worth are based on the evaluation conclusions, let us continue with the example. The evaluators involved the community in the process so the results would be viewed as credible and useful for making any changes deemed necessary to improve access to health care. They used individual interviews and focus groups to collect the qualitative data and incorporated ideas from Appreciative Inquiry so they had some idea of what specific changes to make if necessary. The evaluators incorporated additional questions into the data collection. They wanted to know to which population the information most applied. They collected information on clinic and emergency-room utilization patterns and reviewed all the clinic documents and data bases that had been used to collect information from the clinic and the hospital before the clinic opened.

Two coders coded the data by identifying the themes and highlighting them. The initial themes for the analysis of the qualitative data were identified from the questions but included new themes that emerged while the data were being coded. The themes in the analysis included:

- Knowledge of clinic operations

- Knowledge of clinic services

- Attitudes and behaviors that relate to utilization of the various clinic services

- Perceived improvement in access to health services

- Attitudes toward the use of emergency rooms for nonemergency care

- Knowledge of the policy/policy change that resulted in the opening of the health clinic

- Knowledge of the impact of the new policy (the clinic and other initiatives to address access to health care) on the community

- Knowledge of health-insurance eligibility criteria

- Actions to increase enrollment under the new eligibility

- Problems associated with enrollment

- Problems associated with using the new facilities

- Impact and perceived impact of the new facilities on user groups with different demographics

Major and minor themes were identified to simplify the interpretation of the data.

The coders compared their coding structure after coding the first three transcripts to make sure they were coding items similarly and were clear about the definitions that each had created if a new theme emerged. Because the interviews included men, women, and youth, coders searched for concepts that represented differences in the perceptions of these groups. They organized the data and the analysis to capture any differences. The different responses from clinic users and key informants were identifiable in the sorting and coding because the transcripts were printed on different-colored paper. The coders identified two or three quotes for each of the themes that represented the breadth of the data. The quantitative data were compiled to show utilization patterns before and after the clinic opened using a time-series design. Graphs and tables showed the data pictorially.

The qualitative and the quantitative data together allowed the research question to be answered. The expectation of the objective was that utilization of the emergency room for nonemergency health care would drop by 15 percent, but the evaluation found that it had dropped 20 percent. In addition, the drop was mostly in children who had asthma and used the emergency room because they had no other source of care before the clinic was opened. The data also showed these results:

- Community members were familiar with the new policy and had registered their children so they would have access to nonemergency health care. They had no trouble enrolling their children.

- Community members knew about the clinic and its services from the outreach workers long before the clinic was opened.

- Community members trusted the clinic to provide good care and were satisfied with the care they received twelve months after the clinic opened.

- Community members no longer saw the need to use the emergency room for non-urgent care and praised the staff of the clinic for taking care of them in a timely manner.

- Not all groups utilized the services uniformly. Women and children used the clinic much more than men. Men were still seeking care in the emergency room, and their utilization had not changed in spite of the presence of the clinic.

The information from both the quantitative and the qualitative data was good news for the board of directors and the executive director of the nonprofit organization that had gone to great lengths to understand the problem before opening the clinic. The data showed that the clinic's diversion of people from the emergency room resulted in considerable savings in tax dollars. Triangulation of the data-collection sources and methods allowed the evaluation team to be confident of their findings. They concluded that opening the clinic was valuable to the community. The value was demonstrated in lower costs for the hospital, in lower levels of anxiety for the community, and in greater access to satisfactory nonemergency health services. A win-win situation!

The outreach staff of the clinic were delighted with the conclusion of the evaluation overall, but were concerned that the focus-group data showed that men did not feel they knew enough about the clinic and did not think the clinic provided services for them. The outreach staff pointed this finding out to the executive director, and they developed a plan for increasing the number of men using the clinic. Because they had asked participants for concrete steps for improving the initiative and for shaping systems and relationships differently with the new clinic, they had a lot of information to start with.

THE ROLE OF STAKEHOLDERS

As with quantitative-data analysis and interpretations, stakeholders are usually less involved in this stage of the process; however, qualitative-data analysis is more intuitive than quantitative analysis, and with some training they should be able to learn how to do it. Having stakeholders involved allows the team to check their interpretations of the qualitative data as well as to check their assumptions in observations and other data sources. Stakeholder involvement increases the validity of the findings and increases the likelihood that they will be used.

SUMMARY

- Conducting qualitative research using interviewing approaches—focus groups, individual interviews, Appreciative Inquiry, case studies, digital storytelling, or components of photovoice—provides data that are converted into text through transcription. The resulting document can then be coded to produce themes that form the basis for answering the research questions and drawing conclusions.

- In writing reports, it is important to select quotations that are representative of the theme and that illustrate a shared perception or opinion of the respondents.

(Continued)

(Continued)

Quotations may also be used to highlight particular or interesting phenomena that may form the basis for further research but may not be typical of the views of most of the participants in the study.

▪ Qualitative methods can complement each other to reduce the likelihood of bias and provide a comprehensive understanding of the topic under study.

▪ Conclusions are drawn against the standards including assessing how and whether the process and outcome objectives were met.

DISCUSSION QUESTIONS AND ACTIVITIES

1. Identify a five- to ten-page transcript of a focus-group discussion or an individual interview. Review the transcript and highlight each theme that occurs in a different color. Using a pair of scissors, cut out each theme, keeping a part of the text for quotes and context. Write a summary report of your interview data including quotes. What conclusions would you draw from your results? How might they differ from another person's?

2. Identify a published qualitative study. Review the results of the data collection, and without looking at the authors' interpretation, write up your own interpretations of the data. Compare your interpretation with that of the author. Did they differ? If so, why do you think they did.

3. Review the published literature for evaluations utilizing GIS mapping. How was the method used? What kinds of conclusions was the author able to draw?

KEY TERMS

coding   data-analysis software
computer coding   transcription

CHAPTER

11

REPORTING
EVALUATION FINDINGS

LEARNING OBJECTIVES

- Describe the content of evaluation reports.
- Describe the formats and presentation of evaluation reports.
- Write an evaluation report.

The final step in the Participatory Model for Evaluation is to report the findings (Figure 11.1). A report provides feedback about the results of the evaluation to multiple stakeholder audiences. It describes the evaluation process and findings and makes recommendations in response to the purpose of the evaluation so that the results will be used. Patton (2008, p. 37) defines *utilization-focused evaluation* as "evaluation done for and with the specific intended primary users for specific, intended uses." He goes on to say that the entire evaluation process must be conducted carefully if the evaluation is to be useful. He cautions that the report is only one of many mechanisms for facilitating the use of evaluation findings. Reports nonetheless should communicate information for the benefit of the stakeholders for whom the evaluation was intended. Reports provide feedback on the evaluation questions that were asked and information for both accountability and decision making. They provide necessary and vital accountability not just for the initiative but also for the evaluation team and its stewardship.

As there is no one way to conduct an evaluation, so there is no one way to report the findings. The findings in the report are directly linked to the purpose of the evaluation. For example, if the purpose of the evaluation was to understand the initiative's implementation, then the evaluation approach was a formative or process evaluation. The report would therefore provide information that is helpful for determining whether the initiative was being implemented as planned or whether adjustments were required. Alternatively, if the purpose of the evaluation was to determine the impact of the

FIGURE 11.1.   *The Participatory Framework for Evaluation: Report the Findings*

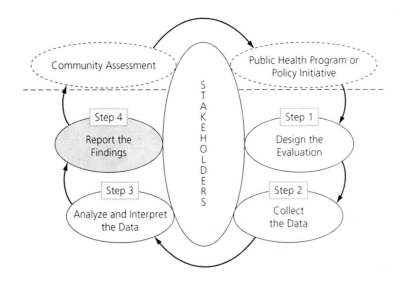

program, both the evaluation approach and the report would provide information on the effect of the program on the beneficiaries. If the purpose of the evaluation was to determine the cost effectiveness of the initiative compared with others, the report would provide a comparison of multiple programs and a level of detail that may not have been necessary or appropriate in reporting a process evaluation.

In addition to keeping the purpose of the evaluation in mind when writing the report, it is helpful to bear in mind the expectations of stakeholders. Stakeholders may have additional expectations, which may include, for example, a discussion of issues of social justice in the report. If stakeholders are involved throughout the process, controversial or potentially difficult conclusions can be discussed. Discussing evaluation findings with stakeholders throughout supports the overall intention of improving the likelihood that the report will be used.

Whether the evaluation is conducted for a public health program or a policy initiative, the value of the process is in the ability of the stakeholders to utilize the findings. There are three major reasons why evaluation results are used:

1. The stakeholders have been involved in the process.

2. The report is written in a user-friendly appropriate format.

3. The results are relevant to stakeholders and provide useful information.

If the real value in conducting an evaluation is in using the findings to improve the program, then the report should report the information in ways that are helpful. The results of evaluations may be used in multiple ways that include revealing new insights into the program and how it works or reordering priorities in program administration or in program direction. The results can lead to a change in the population that is served or to a new direction in policy development. They can result in ending the initiative altogether, or they can persuade stakeholders, policymakers, institutions, professional or civic groups that the initiative is successful. More and more often evaluation is a requirement for further funding, and the report becomes an indispensable tool in raising money and acquiring resources.

Some of these examples may lead one to believe that an evaluation report must provide information only about an initiative's success. Nothing is further from the truth! An evaluation report must answer the research questions in an objective and unbiased way irrespective of positive or negative findings. In general, reports should be understandable, meaningful, valuable, and accurate, and recommendations should be grounded in and reflect the findings from the data (Patton, 2008). It is imperative that report recommendations be within the scope of the agency's work.

This chapter describes the content of the report and suggests formal and alternative ways of providing feedback and the results of the evaluation to a variety of stakeholders. In the Participatory Model for Evaluation, the stakeholder remains central to the process and is a full participant both in the writing of the report and in its delivery.

Evaluation reports must be presented in a manner that facilitates understanding and subsequent use, in a timely way, and by a member of the team, preferably the individual or individuals who have the most credibility with the audience. For example, a youth member of the evaluation team, rather than the team leader, may present the report to the youth who were the subjects of the evaluation because the team leader may have little in common with the group members who should hear and act on the recommendations.

Important considerations in the development of the report are

▪ content

▪ audience

▪ timing

▪ format

Unlike data collected for research purposes in other settings, evaluations are conducted by the evaluation team for and on behalf of an organization, an agency, a foundation, a board of directors, a federal agency, and so forth. The data from the evaluation research and the reports belong to the organization or agency that commissioned the report. Findings from the study and the evaluation report are released to the person or entity that requested the study and are not released without permission to other stakeholders.

THE CONTENT OF THE REPORT

The content of the evaluation report is derived from the data required to support the message that must be conveyed. The information that is provided in the report answering the evaluation questions and supporting the purpose of the evaluation. In addition, the information must be sufficient to clearly describe the program being evaluated, the context, the purposes of the evaluation, the procedures, and the findings (Joint Committee on Standards for Educational Evaluation et al., 1994).

The conclusions of the evaluation describe the value of the initiative to the different stakeholder audiences. The value of the initiative may be both tangible and intangible and is assessed against multiple criteria that include:

▪ The goals and objectives of the initiative as outlined in the evaluation plan

▪ Expectations for what the initiative should achieve

▪ Expectations of who should benefit from the initiative

▪ The reasons for which the evaluation was conducted

▪ Issues of social justice and equity

In addition to being assessed against expected outcomes, the data are also examined for unexpected outcomes that benefit or hurt the community or participants or nonparticipants in the initiative.

The questions for the evaluation may be identified and categorized as major or minor questions, and the findings may be similarly categorized. Major findings may be significant changes that occurred in individuals, community, and systems as a result of the initiative or may be answers to the questions that were selected as most important for the evaluation process. Major findings may also include unintended consequences that had significant impact on individuals, communities, institutions, or systems. Minor findings may be related to less consequential evaluation questions or may be unintended consequences of the intervention.

In writing an evaluation report, use simple, direct language and avoid using jargon and unfamiliar acronyms. Use examples, anecdotes, graphs, charts, diagrams and quotations to illustrate difficult concepts.

The main body of the evaluation report has six key components:

1. Introduction

   ▪ Literature review

   ▪ Community assessment

2. Description of evaluation activities

   ▪ Description of the initiative

   ▪ Evaluation questions

   ▪ Methodology

3. Results and analysis

4. Conclusion and recommendations

5. Limitations and lessons learned

6. Appendix

The Introduction

The introduction to the evaluation report contains a summary of the peer-reviewed scientific literature and published documents that provide information about the distribution, prevalence, incidence, and risk factors associated with the public health problem. It discusses the issue from a national, state, and local perspectives. In addition, the introduction includes a summary of findings from the community assessment. Together they provide the rationale for the development of the initiative.

Description of Evaluation Activities

This section contains a report of the major components of the evaluation. It includes a detailed description of the initiative. The logic model summarizes the initiative's Theory of Change, and the initiative's activities, expected outcomes, outputs, and resources are identified.

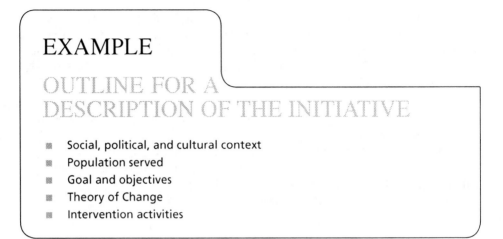

EXAMPLE

OUTLINE FOR A
DESCRIPTION OF THE INITIATIVE

- Social, political, and cultural context
- Population served
- Goal and objectives
- Theory of Change
- Intervention activities

In addition, this section presents the purpose of the evaluation, the evaluation questions, the evaluation plan, and the research design. It discusses stakeholder involvement and roles in the evaluation process.

It provides a detailed description of data-collection strategies, including information about where and how the data were gathered and the analysis was undertaken. The description of the data analysis specifies the software used and the data-analysis and data-management approaches that were included.

The Results

This section discusses the results of the data collection. It contains a description of the sample, summarizes the findings from the quantitative or qualitative data collection, and presents an appropriate analysis and interpretation of the data.

Quantitative data are generally reported in narrative form and are accompanied by charts, tables, graphs, and figures to summarize the data and improve understanding. A summary of the demographic profile of the participants in the sample and an analysis of the survey data are included. For example, if the research question required pre/post–test surveys, then the analysis would include an appropriate comparison. Alternatively, if the question concerned the level of collaboration among members of a coalition, an appropriate representation of the data would be results from a network analysis and a discussion of findings.

Qualitative data are also presented in narrative form, but they are accompanied by quotations or photographs that best represent the theme that is being described. For example, in a recent evaluation study, when the theme being explored was access to health care, a key informant talked in an interview about the difficulties that some people had, one of which was language. This quotation provides powerful imagery for the reader: "Foreign-speaking persons with communication difficulties may have more difficulty in getting care."

The Conclusion

The conclusion of the evaluation report discusses the results of the study in the context of the evaluation criteria. It provides the evaluator's judgment of the initiative overall and a critical assessment of the links among the program inputs, activities, outputs, and outcomes. In addition, it provides a fair and balanced examination of the strengths and weaknesses of the initiative. The judgment associated with the conclusions and hence the recommendations that are made incorporate the results of quantitative and qualitative research with the underlying philosophy of triangulation. Triangulation implies the use of one or more investigators, data sources, or theoretical frameworks in responding to each research question. The results are compared against the standards that have been discussed in previous chapters. They are the standards identified by staff, community members, and program participants. Factors that strengthen the judgment being made include summarizing plausible pathways by which the results could have been reached, suggesting alternative pathways, giving possible reasons why initial objectives and expectations were not supported by the findings of the evaluation, and demonstrating that the results were obtained using systematic and reproducible processes.

The conclusion of an evaluation report

- presents a list of key findings that highlight important aspects of the evaluation results

- reflects on the importance of the findings

- discusses the results of the evaluation in the context of social-justice criteria

- identifies unintended consequences

- suggests other questions that may still need to be answered

- makes recommendations for decision making and stakeholder and community action

The Recommendations

The recommendations are a critical component of the evaluation report. The primary purpose is to communicate actions for consideration by the stakeholders. The actions that are recommended by the evaluation team must be based on the findings from the evaluation process and must be defensible, realistic, and targeted. Recommendations must include not just the recommended actions but reflections on their advantages and disadvantages as well as the cost implications if they are adopted. In addition, Patton (2008, pp. 502–504) identifies political sensitivity, thoughtfulness, and directness as characteristics of recommendations. Recommendations must also support an existing work plan, or be easily incorporated.

For recommendations to be action-oriented they must be specific and considerate of the contextual factors that influence the organization's or agency's operations. For example, a community-based organization's primary activities were to offer

HIV/AIDS prevention and treatment services to youth. Based on an assessment of the objectives of the program, the evaluation team determined that the organization had not met its targets. The evaluators made the following recommendations:

- Increase efforts to reach the target population by increasing outreach and services.

- Increase efforts to improve behavioral risk assessments by the target population by developing mechanisms by which each participant completes the assessment during his or her first visit for prevention case management.

- Continue to explore strategies to implement the curriculum's use through improving links to youth and appropriate communities.

Recommendations may be influenced by the purpose of the evaluation and hence the intended utilization of the findings. The following examples illustrate how findings are linked to the purpose of the evaluation.

- *Purpose:* To understand the extent to which the program is being implemented as planned with a view to expanding to serve a larger population.

- *Finding:* The process evaluation showed that although some parts of the program were well implemented, others lacked sufficient staff support to provide the level of intensity required.

  - Suggest ways that the initiative can realistically increase staffing levels based on the organization's structure and funding, which may necessitate the inclusion of a larger volunteer component.

  - Suggest delaying any expansion of the program until staffing levels are higher.

- *Purpose:* To determine whether the initiative is making or has made an impact on the beneficiaries.

- *Finding:* The outcome evaluation showed that female youth had higher mean scores that were significantly different from those of the male youth.

  - Suggest ways that the initiative can increase the intensity of the offerings for males.

- *Purpose:* To determine the initiative's cost effectiveness compared with that of other programs in an assessment of funding priorities.

- *Finding:* Although the initiative was found to be effective, the cost associated with it was much higher than the cost of similar programs with similar outcomes.

  - Suggest ways of trimming the cost of the initiative without losing the integrity of the initiative.

Limitations, Lessons Learned, and the Appendix

Limitations of the evaluation and *lessons learned* from conducting the evaluation are identified in this section of the report. It describes any shortcomings of the evaluation and reflections on the research approach, participant recruitment, data collection, and research findings. It includes a discussion of the reliability and validity issues that influenced the research and provides an opportunity to discuss improvements in the evaluation process that may be applicable in similar evaluations.

The *appendix* of the evaluation report contains copies of the surveys, consent forms, interview and observation protocols, and similar materials that were used for data collection; it also includes a list of members of the evaluation team and their roles in the evaluation.

THE TIMING OF THE REPORT

There are primarily two times for writing an evaluation report: at the end of the contract period or as an interim report during the period of the evaluation. In both cases the report is presented in time for use. The timing of reports is generally part of the contract that is drawn up at the start of the project. For an outcome evaluation based on a cross-sectional research design, an interim report may be specified in the contract and a final report may be due on completion of the analysis. If the contract period is five years, evaluation reports may be due annually.

In addition, ad hoc reports may be required for decision making at any time during the life of the evaluation contract. This requirement may be negotiated in advance, or the team may be asked to provide a report with some notice. Ad hoc reports may be requested for advisory committee or board meetings, especially in the formative stages of a project or in the case of a process evaluation.

The evaluation report should preferably go to the client at least two weeks before the deadline to allow for adequate reflection and appropriate response and the opportunity for stakeholders to provide input into the recommendations. Allowing sufficient time for review may be especially important when the findings are negative. Participation of the stakeholders in this process will increase the likelihood that the report will be read and used. In an evaluation of a community-based organization, the program manager was given an opportunity to see the final report. As a result, an additional recommendation was included that supported the work of the project manager and provided visibility for the actions that needed to be taken by the organization to meet an important objective. It also ensured that resources would be made available.

THE AUDIENCE FOR THE REPORT

The results of the evaluation are discussed with major stakeholders. The entire evaluation team must participate in this final process. Stakeholders are people who have an interest in knowing the results of the evaluation study, and they constitute the audience for it. These people include:

▓ Program managers and those who commissioned the evaluation

▓ Local, state, and federal policymakers and decision makers

▓ Funding agencies and foundations

▓ Researchers and program developers

▓ Agency board members

▓ Members of the staff and volunteers

▓ Members of the community who are affected by and /or participate in the offerings of the initiative

The audience determines the format of the report, the level of detail in the report, the type of presentation, whether written or oral, and the timing of the report.

THE FORMAT OF THE REPORT

The final evaluation report can have a variety of forms and formats as determined by the purpose of the evaluation and the person(s) requesting or interested in the report and its findings. A report intended for the board of directors will be different from a report for community members. As stakeholders they both are entitled to a presentation of evaluation findings, but they each have separate expectations for the form it should take.

In addition, the selection of the most appropriate format is guided by the characteristics of the initiative, the appropriateness of the format for a particular audience, and its cost. For example, the board of a nonprofit organization or a foundation may expect a formal printed copy of the report complete with an executive summary, while the members of the coalition, who are involved in the day-to-day work of the organization, may prefer a discussion of the main findings with specific recommendations for the actions that are within their control.

Irrespective of the format and whether the evaluation report is in a printed format or will be delivered orally, start by letting the audience know the focus of the report. The title of the report should make the focus clear.

A formal printed version of the report may be developed for a board of directors, advisory committees, funding agencies, or the executive director and contain a number of components.

The *cover page* contains the title, the name of the organization or agency that commissioned the report, the names of the evaluation team members, and the date of the report.

The *table of contents* lists the topics covered in the order they appear in the report and their page numbers.

The *acknowledgments* identify and thank individuals or organizations who contributed to the evaluation, including members of the evaluation team, staff, and participants in the research.

The *list of acronyms* defines short forms and abbreviations of words used in the report that might be unfamiliar to readers.

The *executive summary* is a one- to two-page synopsis of the full report.

The *topics covered* are the background to the evaluation, the evaluation activities, the results, key findings, conclusions, and recommendations.

The final report may be provided in print form in multiple copies or in electronic form on CD or a combination of the two. The contract often defines the format and the timing of the report. In addition to presenting the full report accompanied by the executive summary, an oral and PowerPoint® presentation summarizing the report may be presented to stakeholders.

An oral presentation contains the full report, yet it generally captures the main ideas more succinctly and in more animated and graphic forms. It is generally divided into three parts. The *introduction* sets the tone for the presentation and allows the presenter to get the audience's full attention. The *middle* explains the evaluation and presents the results of the study. The *end* provides the recommendations, discusses the next steps, and leaves the audience with a set of specific recommended actions.

If, however, the evaluation report is being developed for members of the community, more appropriate and less formal approaches must be developed. The final report format and content may also be negotiated with stakeholders.

The format and the content of the less formal presentations will depend on the community or stakeholder group. Important considerations include reading levels, involvement in the process, and the extent to which recipients understand what the evaluation was about. The more engaged stakeholders are in the evaluation, the more likely they are to grasp the details of the research design and the data-collection approach. The format must also be culturally appropriate. In addition, when reports are for youth audiences, using youth-appropriate media is vital.

Appropriate formats for a range of audiences include the following:

- Full report of the evaluation approaches, methodology, findings, recommendations, and conclusions

- One- to two-page executive summary of the full report

- Single-page summary of the major findings and recommendations

- Press releases

- Newspaper-, newsletter-, magazine-, or brochure-style reports highlighting the main findings and recommendations with a focus on what members of the community can do to address the problem

- Community presentations in town hall meetings highlighting the main findings and presenting recommendations that the community can act on immediately and in the long term

- Graphic and/or animated digital-media or radio or television presentations highlighting important findings

- Media presentations that allow the evaluation team to not only present the report but also to discuss its implications with stakeholder groups

- Oral presentations that highlight the main findings and provide audiences the opportunity to ask questions and to clarify conclusions

- Photographs

Additionally, presentations of evaluation findings may occur at conferences and meetings where formal oral, PowerPoint®, and poster presentations may be made summarizing the full report. Technical reports and journal articles may also be used to support academic writings. An abstract is usually required for academic writings. An abstract consists of

- the background—a brief overview of the purpose of the evaluation

- the numbers, location, and demographic characteristics of participants

- the design of the study and an overview of type of data collected

- the results of qualitative and/or quantitative research

- the conclusions and recommendations for next steps

Irrespective of the format that is used, the reporting of evaluation results should

- be accurate

- match the culture and reading levels of the audience

- provide an appropriate level of detail so the audience understands the approach, the findings, and the recommendations

- include illustrations, examples, and quotations that provide depth to the data and improve the authenticity of the report

- communicate respect and fairness to the audience

- provide the audience with clear action-oriented next steps

- use well-designed and effective presentations

- involve stakeholders throughout the process

Ultimately the evaluation report is a two-way communication between the evaluation team and the stakeholders. The evaluation team ensures that the results are understood; stakeholders get a chance to ask questions; and the evaluation team guides them to implement the recommendations and prepare for the next evaluation cycle.

SUMMARY

- Stakeholders must be involved in the development of the report and recommendations as they were throughout the process.

- Evaluation results are used when the stakeholders have been involved in the process, the report is written in a user-friendly, appropriate format, and, most important, the results are relevant to stakeholders and provide useful information.

- The evaluation report contains an explanation of the research study, results, analysis, and recommendations. It includes major and significant findings as well as minor, less consequential findings. It includes a discussion of unintended consequences that had a significant impact on individuals, communities, institutions, or systems, and it discusses issues of social justice.

- The selection of the format for the final presentation and report is guided by the characteristics of the initiative; the information to be provided; the audiences for the report; the delivery channels (print, electronic, in person); and the cost.

- The reporting of evaluation results should be accurate, be appropriate for the culture and reading levels of the audience, include an appropriate level of detail, and use illustrations, examples, and quotations that provide depth to the findings and improve the authenticity of the report.

- The report must communicate respect and fairness to the audience and provide the audience with clear action-oriented next steps

DISCUSSION QUESTIONS AND ACTIVITIES

1. You are part of an evaluation team that has just completed a three-year study of a local community organization's initiatives with a lot of findings. What factors would you take into consideration in preparing the final report? What would be the most appropriate venue for your presentation of the evaluation findings?

2. Identify evaluation findings for a public health initiative. Report the findings in a format suitable for a low-literacy community group. How would you disseminate your report?

3. In preparing an evaluation report of a youth intervention, what approaches would you select? Develop a multimedia presentation for this audience.

KEY TERMS

evaluation findings
evaluation report

executive summary
presentation formats

CASE STUDY

Note: The names and data used in this case study are made up and do not refer to any existing persons or situations.

THE COMMUNITY ASSESSMENT

Background

The number of persons with diabetes has increased steadily over the past decade. During that time, diabetes has been one of the leading causes of death, and heart disease is often associated with it. Diabetes-associated cardiovascular disease is the largest component of the direct costs of hospitals. Diabetes is a major clinical and public health challenge.

There were high rates of diabetes in a rural community of 250,000 people in Riverside County, and many people had lost limbs because of diabetes-related amputations. Community members wanted to know about the condition, and a team was assembled to conduct a community assessment.

Establish a Team

The team was a demographically diverse group of fifteen people who mostly lived or worked or both in the community. A few people on the team who did not live or work there knew the community well because they had done work with some of the local groups a few years before. But they had stayed in touch with the community and loved to come back for celebrations.

The team agreed on the task. They would conduct a community assessment to understand why this community had such high rates of diabetes, but more than that they wanted to know how to improve community health. The group went around the table and said their names and why they wanted to be there. The project coordinator realized it was a diverse group and decided that a team-building exercise would be a good start. The exercise focused on building an understanding of each other's cultures.

The team adapted an activity from a book about building evaluation capacity. The group discussed how language, food and eating, learning and information processing, the concept of time, communication styles, relationships, individual and community values and norms, work habits, and other practices influence work in general and evaluation in particular. It was a spirited conversation, which helped clarify misconceptions about others' cultures.

After the team-building activities, the team took a short break and then reassembled to discuss the task before them. They felt they could contribute to the community assessment. The project director had come across a definition of cultural competence that she liked and wanted to share it: "A set of congruent behaviors, attitudes, and policies that come together in a system, agency, or among professionals and enables that system, agency, or those professionals to work effectively in cross-cultural situations." After the training, the group adopted the definition of competence as a goal for the team. One of the members introduced a game that allowed people to talk about their skills in a nonthreatening way and appreciate the value of each person's contribution to the team. They discovered that they had many skills and talents among them and much in common; and they all felt they had a lot to contribute to the process. Their skills and talents are summarized in Table 12.1; they included:

TABLE 12.1. Potential Contributions of Team Members

Members	Potential Contributions
Project coordinator	Project management, study design, field testing instruments, analyzing and interpreting qualitative data
Community members representing churches, schools, women's groups	Instrument design, data collection, reviewing and interpreting qualitative- and quantitative-analysis results
Staff of state agencies, local government departments, and community-based organizations	Instrument design, data collection, analyzing qualitative and quantitative data
Researcher	Study design, instrument design, analyzing and interpreting quantitative and qualitative data

- Experience in writing simple proposals and budgets

- Experience with conducting interviews and collecting surveys. One person had used photovoice before and found it helpful for engaging more people and understanding the community perspective.

- Experience in analyzing qualitative and quantitative data

- Experience in project management

The team members spent some time getting to know one another and working as a team. The project coordinator had experience working in teams, and although some of the members had been in meetings together before, they had not worked on the same team. The team-building exercises emphasized respect for each other and valuing each other's cultures and contributions to the project. The team wanted to infuse the Community-Based Participatory Research principles into the process. They especially wanted to make sure they built on the strengths and resources of the community, facilitated collaboration among all group members, and developed a learning community that emphasized capacity building.

Determine the Availability of Data

The first major task for the team was to ascertain what data were already available nationally. One of the members of the team volunteered to conduct a literature review and came back to the group with a short summary.

> There are two major types of diabetes. Type 1, which occurs because of the failure of the body to produce insulin, and Type 2, which results when the body is unable to use the insulin it produces or when the insulin that is present is inefficient. Prediabetes occurs when the levels of glucose in the blood are higher than normal but not high enough to produce a diagnosis of Type 2 diabetes. The risk for Type 2 diabetes increases with age and being a member of a minority population (Jackson et al., 2008). Other risks of diabetes include having diabetes during pregnancy, having high blood pressure, and having high cholesterol levels caused primarily by consuming too much saturated fat and too few vegetables, fruits, and grain products that are high in vitamins and minerals, carbohydrates (starch and dietary fiber), and other substances that are important to good health (Hanity, 2009; Vandam 2008). In addition, being sedentary and not participating in regular exercise are also considered risk factors. Although obesity occurs among all population groups, obesity is most common among African American women (Jones, 2009).

The team members understood how to focus their community assessment. They wanted to understand

- who was most affected by the disease in their community and how they were affected

- how people's diets affect their health

- people's perceptions of the connections among diet, obesity, and health

- people's knowledge, attitudes, and behavior with regard to diabetes, obesity, exercise, general health care, and utilizing health care

- environmental factors that influence the availability of fresh fruits and vegetables and opportunities for exercise

- cultural factors that influence food intake and exercise

- resources available in the community to address the issue

- factors influenced by history, and issues of social justice, and equity

Decide on the Data-Collection Approaches and Methods

Team members decided to organize their study around a theory so it would be easier to design an intervention later. They especially liked the ecological model because it allowed them to consider the factors that influenced diabetes at the individual, interpersonal, community, organizational, and policy levels. They wanted to be more specific than the ecological model allowed, so they included constructs from the Health Belief Model: perceived susceptibility, perceived seriousness of the condition, and barriers to and benefits of addressing the problem. They also used the stages of change from the Transtheoretical Model. Social Cognitive Theory was included to provide constructs of reciprocal determinism, outcome expectations, self-efficacy, self-regulation, and self-efficacy.

Data-Collection Approach   The team members decided that they had a lot to learn. They had skills in both qualitative and quantitative methods, so they focused their attention on the best approaches for getting the information they needed. They understood their population. Most of the women had completed high school, but only a few (1 percent) had gone to college. They gathered regularly for celebrations and were community oriented. They loved to talk and wanted to be involved in everything that was going on in the community. These characteristics were useful for collecting qualitative data. The team also worked with the local hospital and clinics to get data. They would also get a chance to triangulate their findings, making them more valid. They decided to use surveys to collect data that were easily categorized and put into numerical format, but they also decided to use individual interviews and digital stories with accompanying photographs. Stories would be dictated by women who had diabetes and who lived with the consequences of poor access to and utilization of health care; their perspectives would add a dimension that the other methods would not have included. GIS maps were drawn of the area with demographic and diabetes information.

Data-Collection Instruments   The survey was organized into four major sections and a demographic section. The team identified previous surveys that they thought would be useful and adopted some of the questions. And they developed some of their own to create a fifty-item survey that included yes/no and scale-type items. Part 1 of the survey asked about women's diets and their perceptions of the connections among diet, obesity, and health. Part 2 asked about their knowledge, attitudes, and behavior with regard to diabetes, obesity, exercise, general health care, and utilizing health care. Part 3 asked questions that tried to get at cultural factors such as body image, family, community, and socialization and how these factors affected food intake and exercise behaviors and patterns. Part 4 focused on environmental factors that possibly affected access to fresh fruits and vegetables and to exercise. Part 5 included socioeconomic and demographic items, such as age, race, education, marital status, number of children in the household, income, and employment status. African American adult women ages eighteen to sixty were asked to complete the surveys.

Individual key-informant interviews were used primarily to understand the resources available in the community to address the issue and the environmental factors related to access to fresh fruits and vegetables and exercise facilities. In addition, the interviewer solicited information on the history and leadership of the community as well as issues of social justice and equity.

The survey was tested in a pilot study of thirty women who lived in a comparable, nearby community and had similar demographics. Two individual interviews were conducted to pilot the key-informant interview guide. The pilot test included testing the use of the consent form.

Data-Collection Plan   Interviews were scheduled for a time and place that ensured both confidentiality and safety. Surveys took on average twenty minutes to complete, and interviews lasted approximately one hour. Completing the surveys and participating in the in-depth interviews and digital stories were entirely voluntary. Individuals were not compensated for their time.

Training

Members of the research team were trained to serve as interviewers for the individual in-depth interviews through an interactive program that included a discussion of the content and rationale of the study and procedures for documenting participants' responses in the individual interviews. Training gave an overview of the entire research project and an opportunity for participants to provide input into the process and to practice interviewing skills. Training was also provided in using the equipment for digital stories. Facilitators who would administer the surveys were also provided an orientation so as to be able to provide accurate information to the community if questions arose about the purpose of the study and the intended use of the data.

Resource Procurement

Members of the team included members of community-based organizations and state agencies that had some funding for research, so they pooled their resources. They had sufficient money to pay for travel and supplies. The agencies provided in-kind support that covered the production of all the surveys.

Analysis and Interpretation of the Data

The survey data were analyzed using traditional descriptive statistics. Data was presented using traditional graphs along with GIS maps. GIS maps showed the distribution of diabetes across the community using data from the hospital and community health-center records and community resources. The prepared maps could then be compared with maps of poverty, unemployment, occupational structure, educational attainment, household structure, and income to explore the association between diabetes and adverse socioeconomic conditions. The overlay of maps as described suggested potential social, economic, and other risk factors for diabetes and aided in the selection and development of intervention activities.

The data from the digital stories and the individual interviews were analyzed to identify the themes using theoretical and empirical constructs from the literature and embedded in the instruments used for data collection. The qualitative software package NVivo® was used to code the qualitative-data transcripts.

Summary of Findings

The community assessment found that the rates of diabetes among black females who had not completed high school were higher than the rates for white and Hispanic women, with women between the ages of forty and sixty-four being the most affected. The number of new cases of diabetes that year was 6.9 per thousand, a jump from 5.9 per thousand in the previous year. Furthermore, the number of obese women had also increased; 30 percent of women had a BMI greater than 30. A further assessment of risk factors associated with the rates of diabetes in this population included low levels of knowledge about diabetes, its causes, and prevention; poor attitudes about healthy eating and regular exercise; a media market that promoted fast foods. Women described their love of traditional food, which has high levels of saturated fat. The digital stories revealed how much women regretted that they had not paid sufficient attention to their diets and exercise.

This community was what one could call a food desert; only one of the ten convenience stores within the community sold fruits and vegetables at affordable prices. Most of the respondents were not within walking distance of grocery stores, which were on average three miles away. In addition, there were very few affordable exercise facilities.

THE INTERVENTION

Background

There were at least three organizations in the community that provided services. One of them, the Community Action Partnerships for Health Organization (CAPHO), was eager to expand its work to include diabetes. CAPHO had been providing services to low-income African American women for ten years, and they also had noticed the increasing numbers of women who were diagnosed with diabetes in the previous year.

Based on the mission of the organization to "reduce the rates of chronic disease among women who live in the state," they decided they would intervene after they found out the results of the community assessment. The executive director invited her staff to a meeting to assess the organization's capacity to offer an additional service to women. They did a Strengths, Weakness, Opportunities, and Threats (SWOT) analysis to determine the organization's administrative capacity and also to think about the internal and external difficulties that might arise. Once the process was complete, they agreed that although it would stretch their budget, they were already doing some similar interventions as part of other programs. They just needed to add a few new components.

Because they wanted to stay focused on prevention, they decided the goal would be to "reduce the rates of diabetes among low-income African American women in Riverside County." The executive director discussed the proposal with the board of directors, and it was approved. The organization contacted their community advisory committee, which included women in their other programs and staff in other nearby organizations, to discuss their new project. After many meetings, the advisory committee formulated the focus of their prevention program, which would be offered to African American women, the majority of whom were concentrated in three contiguous zip code areas. They decided they would address two important risk factors for the onset of diabetes: obesity and lack of exercise. They talked with the stakeholders and eventually agreed on the scope of the work and the main overarching question for the intervention they called the Healthy Soon Project: "What effect did the Healthy Soon Project have on women who participated?"

The Healthy Soon Project

There were program pieces of the initiative that CAPHO could do in-house, like provide exercise equipment, but they also wanted women to walk around their neighborhoods to the park, to the stores, and just for pleasure with their friends. They recognized that in the low-income communities women had limited opportunities to walk. The sidewalks were broken, the park was unsafe, and grocery stores were too far away for a leisurely stroll. The one convenience store that sold fruits and vegetables often kept them in a box under the counter or in the refrigerator too long. The team would need to get some other folks into the committee who would work on the policy-development component of the initiative. They had their work cut-out for them.

The team did lots of research to help guide them and the expertise around the table also helped. By incorporating the principles of the ecological model, they were able to address more than one level of influence. To factors at the individual level, they added environmental factors that had been identified in the community assessment. The CAPHO team outlined a set of outcome objectives that provided the direction for the development of the project (and could be used as well later as benchmarks for the evaluation).

Public Health Goal: To reduce the rates of diabetes among low-income African American women in Riverside County.

Program Health Objective: Increase the percentage of African American women who participate in the intervention who are at a healthy weight to 60 percent by 2012.

Program Environmental Objective: Increase to 40 percent the number of stores and other venues that sell affordable produce in low-income neighborhoods by 2015.

The assumption made by the team was that with physical activity and good nutrition women would attain and maintain a healthy weight that would lead to a lower incidence and reduced rates of diabetes within the population. Figure 12.1 illustrates this Theory of Change.

The team decided to meet once a week until they had the program clearly planned; then they would meet monthly to check in with each other. They set a deadline for launching the program within six months. By this time they expected they would have allocated or secured the resources for the program.

The team members wanted to use an evidence-based intervention for their program because they knew that such initiatives were likely to be successful. They first broke down each of the objectives to identify the kinds of outcomes they wanted to see and the types of activities they thought would be appropriate for their population of low-income African American women. The literature suggested that African American women prefer to exercise with their friends and families rather than do it by themselves. The team also knew from going into the convenience stores that there was a lot of advertising for alcohol, and women on the committee said that was one reason they discouraged their children from going to the local convenience stores. They thought it was important for the young people to develop better eating habits. One way to do that would be to make the stores more child-friendly.

The team conducted a literature search to identify evidence-based programs or evidence-based principles for nutrition and physical-activity programs. They wanted to determine

- whether any interventions had been tested among low-income African American women

FIGURE 12.1. *Theory of Change*

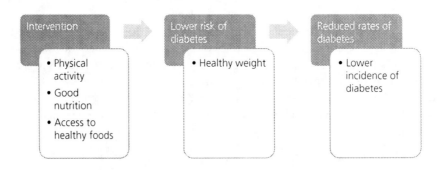

- whether any interventions included weight loss or maintaining a healthy weight or a similar outcome

- whether CAPHO had the human, material, and financial resources needed

The team was able to find recommendations from the American Diabetes Association; the National Institutes of Diabetes, Digestive and Kidney Diseases; and the U.S. Diabetes Prevention Program. The recommendations supported what they wanted to do and gave them additional ideas for activities.

Recommendations included:

- Screening for those who are overweight; are over forty-five years; have a family history of diabetes and high blood pressure; and belong to a minority racial group

- Weight loss with a reduced intake of fat; increased intake of dietary fiber; fewer calories

- Physical activity of moderate intensity for 150 minutes per week

So, they had what they needed for the first objective but did not have anything for the second objective. They had to find out whether there were evidence-based principles for increasing the number of convenience stores that sold fruits and vegetables and what policy changes would support such an initiative. A search of the literature did not turn up much information, but they knew from conferences they had attended that people around the country were developing projects similar to theirs. They contacted some organizations around the country to find out what they had done.

The team constructed a table (Table 12.2) that showed the program goals, the expected outcomes, and the intervention approaches.

As they developed the initiative, they wrote sub-objectives to reflect proximal benchmarks; and the activity objectives supported the outcome objectives. The team was reminded that activities for the initiative had to meet certain criteria. They had to

- lead to the change specified in the objective

- be completed during the specified time frame

- have sufficient resources and personnel

- be appropriate for the culture and expectations of the population for whom they were intended

- be part of an overall plan to achieve a program's goal

With that set of reminders the team got to work. See what they did to develop the outcome objectives in Tables 12.3 and 12.4.

With the help of the evaluation experts described in the next section, the team developed a logic model so they could clarify the initiative (Table 12.5).

TABLE 12.2. **Program Goals, Expected Outcomes, and Intervention Approaches**

Expected Outcome	Intervention Approach
Increase the percentage of African American women who participate in the intervention who are at a healthy weight to 60 percent by 2012.	
Healthy weight (BMI >19 <27)	Nutrition education; healthy diet; peer-supported and in-gym physical activity and monitoring; increased access to fresh fruits and vegetables
Increase to 40 percent the number of stores and other venues that sell affordable produce in low-income neighborhoods by 2015.	
Affordable produce	Convenience stores and farmers' markets; laws and policies that support access to affordable healthy foods in underserved neighborhoods; advocates whose primary focus was increasing access to and availability of food

DESIGN THE EVALUATION

CAPHO's projects had been successful in the past, but this time they wanted to be sure they were reaching their goal, so they discussed bringing an evaluation team in early; by doing so they would be sure to collect the data for the evaluation from the beginning.

A member of the community who had worked with a local community-based organization (CBO) and had been part of their evaluation team suggested Antoinette Pattercake. She was contacted and asked whether she would be available to conduct the study. Just to be sure she would work well with the stakeholders, the team asked her to meet them and provide information about her background, experience, and expertise in conducting evaluations. They were interested in knowing her approach to evaluation and were particularly interested in her ability to work with multiple stake-holders and conduct a participatory evaluation in which they played a major role. They wanted to have a thorough understanding of evaluation when it was all over, so the next time they would feel comfortable taking on their own evaluation studies. Antoinette had her own team of three evaluators who had worked together for five

TABLE 12.3. **Outcome Objectives and Initiative Activities for Healthy-Weight Goal**

Outcome Objective	Initiative Activities	Frequency
Increase the proportion of African American women who participate in the intervention who are at a healthy weight to 60 percent by 2012.		
80 percent of participants in the Healthy Soon Project will report consuming a recommended diet consistently within six weeks of joining the program.	Dietician develops low-fat, high-fiber, low-calorie diets for each participant	Monthly
	Participants keep a diary of food intake and problem solving that reflects struggles in controlling diet and exercising regularly	Daily
	Weigh-ins/testimonials and support groups/discussion of how advertising influences food choices	Bi-monthly
80 percent of participants in the Healthy Soon Project will report exercising for a 150 minutes per week within eight weeks of joining the program.	Recruit friends and family as exercise partners	Daily
	Strength and toning exercise activities	
	Participants keep a diary of duration of exercise	
80 percent of participants in the Healthy Soon Project will maintain prediabetes levels for fasting plasma glucose for one year.	Conduct screenings to monitor fasting plasma glucose levels	Monthly

years. She told the group about them and invited members of the community to join the team. Antoinette and her team used the Participatory Model for Evaluation to guide their work.

Before Antoinette's company, Quality Evaluation Inc., took on the task, they developed a scope-of-work document outlining a plan for an evaluation that would be

TABLE 12.4. **Outcome Objectives and Initiative Activities for Affordable-Produce Goal**

Objective	Initiative Activities	Time Frame
Increase to 40 percent the number of stores that sell affordable produce in low-income neighborhoods by 2015.		
80 percent of local government officials will support the need to increase access to fresh fruits and vegetables in communities by 2012.	Educate policymakers through face-to-face meetings, information brochures, and just-in-time information about the value of having convenience stores sell fresh fruits and vegetables Build a grass-roots coalition to support food security	Monthly
By 2012 25 percent more stores will successfully manage fresh produce.	Train store owners in produce management, business management Provide mentoring for store owners Provide incentives to offset the cost of the program to store owners Build programs that encourage purchase of fruits and vegetables—e.g., buy one, get one free; discount coupons	Ongoing
By 2014 a bill will be passed that provides incentives and other support for carrying fresh foods in convenience stores.	Educate policymakers through face-to-face meetings, information brochures, and just-in-time information	Monthly
By 2014 a policy will be enacted to reduce the height and number of alcohol-related signs in convenience stores.	Work with store owners to reduce the number and height of advertising for alcohol in local stores	Weekly

TABLE 12.5.   **The Logic-Model Components and Healthy Soon Project Activities**

Logic-Model Component	Healthy Soon Project
Resources (inputs)	$150,000 budget for year 1 One supervisor and three support staff Gym facilities Diabetes screening supplies Dietician on contract Farmers
Activities	Nutrition education Low-calorie/low-fat/high-fiber diet Glucose monitoring and weigh-ins/food journaling/strength and toning/walking Farmers' market/fresh fruits and vegetables Educate policymakers Enact legislation to reduce advertising for alcohol in convenience stores Coalition to support access to healthy-foods legislation Work with store owners to reduce advertising for alcohol Train store owners in produce and business management Mentoring for store owners Incentives to store owners and customers Community education on risk factors for diabetes
Outputs	African American women participating in nutrition and exercise components Family members recruited as walking buddies Farmers participating Development of farmers' markets Local store owners trained and fresh-produce sections developed Satisfaction of store owners, farmers, and project participants Legal and regulatory frameworks developed CAPHO/farmers/store owners partnership developed
Expected outcomes (effects)	Knowledge of risk factors for diabetes Increase in the number of stores and other venues that manage and sell fruits and vegetables Increased consumption of dietician-recommended diets Exercising for 105 minutes per week Women maintaining prediabetes levels for fasting glucose Policy enacted to reduce the level and number of alcohol-related advertisements Women maintaining healthy weight (BMI >19<27)

within CAPHO's budget. They wanted to stay within a $50,000 limit. Antoinette knew that would not be a large evaluation, but her evaluators were excited that they would get the chance to do it and to work closely with members of the community. They developed a very modest proposal and planned to keep it small but to make sure that for the first year the questions they would be asking would be, "Was the initiative implemented as planned?" "Was the intended population participating as planned?" They intended to write a grant for funding the evaluation in subsequent years. They decided to use the first year to develop and test some tools and to collect lots of information to serve as the baseline in addition to conducting the process evaluation. Once the contract was signed, they recruited members of the community to join them. They ended with a team of ten members. Some of them had participated in the community assessment, so they were clearly motivated to see their project come to fruition.

It was a great team with a lot of enthusiasm. Antoinette and her evaluators attended their first meeting two weeks later, and by asking many questions they found out about the community's concerns. The evaluators tried to understand the fears expressed by the stakeholders and the steps that had been taken to address them.

The purpose of the evaluation was primarily to gain insight into the program's implementation and Theory of Change, identify any barriers and facilitators to the women's participation, and suggest mid-term corrections if necessary. The initiative's Theory of Change postulated that " if African American women participate in the prescribed nutrition and exercise intervention for a period of six weeks and continue the regimen for at least one year, they will reduce their risk of getting diabetes." The evaluation would determine whether the program had sufficient intensity to achieve this outcome.

Evaluation Questions

The next step was to use the items from the logic model (Table 12.5) as the framework for stakeholders to think about their questions. As a reminder, Antoinette put the logic model on the wall.

Another member of the group, Kingstee, facilitated the session. The evaluators had two major criteria for identifying questions: they had to clearly state what the stakeholder wanted to know, and they had to link directly to the initiative. The group identified thirty evaluation questions. The program was new, so although they had a combination of process and outcome evaluation questions, they focused on understanding whether the program was being implemented appropriately. Kingstee used the nominal technique to narrow them down to seven and then used a two-by-two table (Figure 12.2) to determine which ones the group considered the most important.

These were the seven questions the group identified:

1. What human, financial, and material resources were provided and used?

2. What educational activities were carried out?

FIGURE 12.2. *Two-by-Two Table*

Ability to provide understanding of the critical components of program implementation

	High	Low
High	• Were all the components of the plan implemented? • What is the level of implementation of the women's nutrition and exercise initiatives? • What activities have taken place to support the policy to reduce advertisements for alcohol? • What is the knowledge of diabetes risk factors among women who participate in the initiative?	• What human, financial, and material resources were provided and used?
Low	• What educational activities were carried out?	• What activities have taken place to develop the farmers' market?

Ability to contribute to decision making

3. Were all the components of the plan implemented?

4. What is the level of implementation of the women's nutrition and exercise initiatives?

5. What activities have taken place to develop the farmers' market?

6. What activities have taken place to support the policy to reduce advertisements for alcohol?

7. What is the knowledge of diabetes risk factors among women who participate in the initiative?

The evaluation team wanted answers to two additional questions:

1. Are the data-collection tools appropriate for assessing program outcomes?

2. Do preliminary findings indicate that the intervention is likely to produce the anticipated outcomes?

As a result of this exercise the evaluation team focused on the five questions in the top part of the table. Answering these questions would most likely provide the information they needed to determine whether the critical components of the program were being implemented appropriately. Although the other questions were important, the team had a limited budget, so they had to identify the most important questions, the ones that were critical to the Theory of Change.

Because the evaluation started early in the program's development, the appropriate type of evaluation would be a formative evaluation, that appears to also be the focus of stakeholders' concerns. Process-evaluation questions are similar to formative-evaluation questions. The difference is that process evaluation is used when the program is more stable than it is when it is being developed, which is when formative evaluation is appropriate. The questions were sorted into formative and outcome questions (Table 12.6) so everybody would be clear about what was being done and to help members of the team learn about evaluation.

Formative and process evaluations assess the context, the reach, the dosage, or the intensity of the initiative and the fidelity with which it is delivered. They assess the initiative at the level of resources/inputs and outputs and determine the effectiveness of the administrative functions of the program. Process and outcome evaluations confirm the Theory of Change in mature programs. Quality monitoring continues throughout the project.

Indicators and Data Sources

The next task for the team was to develop the indicator table to show what measures would be required (Table 12.7).

TABLE 12.6.   Evaluation Questions

Formative	Outcome
Were all the components of the plan implemented?	What is the knowledge of diabetes risk factors among women who participate in the initiative?
What is the level of implementation of the women's nutrition and exercise initiatives?	
What activities have taken place to support the policy to reduce advertisements for alcohol?	
What human, financial, and material resources were provided and used?	

TABLE 12.7.   **Indicators and Data Sources**

Evaluation Question	Indicator	Source of Data
Were all the components of the plan implemented?	Women participating in nutrition and exercise interventions Family and friends recruited as walking buddies Development of farmers' markets Local store owners trained and fresh produce sections developed Satisfaction of store owners, farmers, and project participants Legal and regulatory frameworks developed CAPHO/farmers/store owners partnership developed, number of stores/farmers' markets	Attendance logs Minutes from meetings Training reports Record reviews Observation Site visits
What is the level of implementation of the women's nutrition and exercise initiatives?	Number or meetings with dietician Number of sessions per week in the gym Number of walks with family member per day Number of bi-monthly screenings Food diaries/journal entries of quality/quantity of food	Site visits Interviews with staff and participants Laboratory reports Record reviews Food diary/journal reviews Observation
What activities have taken place to support the policy to reduce advertisements for alcohol?	Number of monthly information sessions/ newsletters/e-mails to policymakers Number of participants in grass-roots coalition Number and type of actions by coalition members to educate/advocate	Copies of materials Attendance logs E-mail lists Minutes from meetings

(Continued)

TABLE 12.7.   *(Continued)*

Evaluation Question	Indicator	Source of Data
What human, financial, and material resources were provided and used?	Program in place Personnel hired Space utilized Laboratory invoices $ Purchase receipt $	Record review Audit Attendance records Meeting minutes Data-base review Interview with accounting staff Observation
What is the knowledge of diabetes risk factors among women who participate in the initiative?	Percentage increase in number of people with knowledge of diabetes	Survey

Ensuring the Quality of the Evaluation

The Quality Evaluation Inc. team discussed the overall research design to assess whether they would be able to determine that the intervention had made a difference. They went back to the project documents and saw that the Healthy Soon intervention would last for six weeks and then the women would be expected to continue exercising on their own and following the diet plan. They would continue having their weigh-ins and screenings and completing their journals for a year. Therefore, the design they would use to determine the effect of the program was a pre/post quasi-experimental design with a second posttest one year after the women had completed the initial six-week intervention. They were delighted that they had been called into the initiative early enough to collect baseline data and to make sure there was sufficient documentation of the activities. They could then be confident that the intervention had caused the changes they were observing.

The women who joined the program were selected randomly from a pool of women who were eligible for the program. CAPHO advertised the program using fly-ers, announcements in local churches, at day care centers, and so forth; they had women register to participate in the Healthy Soon Project. After three weeks they randomly assigned fifty people from the list to be in the intervention group. Another fifty were randomly assigned to be in the comparison group. The evaluation team was trying to avoid a biased sample. When they compared the two groups later, they found that they were similar, so they had done a good job in the selection process.

Because the women in the comparison group had the same risk factors for diabetes, the program wanted to compensate them for their time. In addition, they wanted to help them reduce their risk of diabetes by offering them a reduced intervention. The comparison group got: (1) a single one-hour lecture on diabetes, screening tests, a six-month weigh-in, and they were asked to complete a journal recording any exercise they took and their daily meals; and (2) a free membership to the gym in the second year. Both groups got transportation vouchers whenever they came in for screening.

The evaluators had to also make sure they minimized the threats to internal validity. See Table 12.8 for the steps they took.

COLLECT THE DATA

The evaluation team spent some time discussing how they would use their time profitably to collect all the information they needed. To facilitate the training of team members, each established member of Quality Evaluations Inc. mentored two new members. Mentoring required their working closely with their mentees and teaching them what they were doing. Mentees had to do more than observe; they had books to read and worksheets to complete. By completing the worksheets together, the team knew what information they would need to gather and how they would do it.

The next task was to develop the tools for data collection. For example, the team needed to develop data bases so all the information with regard to expenditure and participation were entered. They also wanted to be able to keep a running tally of e-mails that went out to coalition members. Tools had to be developed in this way for each of the indicators.

The team provided training to all the staff so they understood the importance of data collection and how to complete all the tools. Training was provided on how to enter data in the data base. The data base would be used to track everything: the women's participation, their laboratory results, their weights, and the intensity of their exercise. The data base would be useful for answering the second question that the team had: "Do preliminary findings indicate that the intervention is likely to produce the anticipated outcomes?"

Tools developed for ongoing monitoring included:

- A site-visit report
- Journal entries
- An attendance sheet
- A record review sheet

In addition to completing the process evaluation and developing tools for ongoing monitoring, the evaluation team developed some additional materials that they would use as part of the outcome evaluation. One was an interview and the other was a pre/post–test survey.

TABLE 12.8.   **Addressing Threats to Internal Validity**

Threat to Validity	Actions of the Evaluation Team
Attrition: The loss of participants in the intervention	Participants will be told the importance of their participation and encouraged to participate with the use of incentives during and following their successful completion of the six-week and one-year evaluations.
History: Events that take place outside the intervention	Participants will include information in their journals about anything they did or heard that was different from the intervention and that would likely change the nature of the intervention for some people and not for others.
Instrumentation: Changes that occur to the reliability and validity of measurement tools	The evaluation team will ensure that all the data-collection instruments are reliable and valid.
Maturation: Changes in the study participants caused by natural and physiological changes	The women who participate in this intervention will grow older and more experienced during the year they participate in the intervention. These changes will occur in all participants at different levels.
Regression: The study participants are selected on the basis of high or low baseline scores	The team will ensure high reliability in testing and will be sure that no individual's scores are much higher or much lower than the population mean scores.
Selection: Differences in the study population between the intervention and the comparison group	The team will use randomly selected groups for both the intervention and the comparison groups to ensure their equivalence. In addition they will compare the groups using statistical tests to determine that they were in fact similar.
Statistical-Conclusion Validity: The sample size is too small to show the effect	The sample size will be sufficiently large to reduce the threat. Evaluators will ensure that their instruments are reliable to reduce errors in measurement and will try to ensure standard delivery of the intervention to all participants. The journal entries and staff logs will help track these precautions.
Testing: Changes that occur to participants as a result of the number of times they are tested	Evaluators will not provide participants with the correct responses to the multiple-choice test at the baseline, and participants will not get their responses back. In addition, although the same questions will be on the posttest, the order of the responses will be changed.

TABLE 12.9.   **Sample Site-Visit Report**

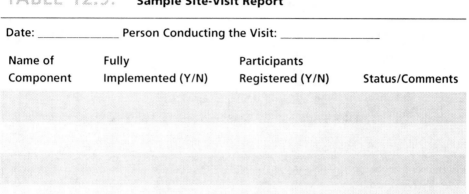

Date: _____ Person Conducting the Visit: _____

Name of Component	Fully Implemented (Y/N)	Participants Registered (Y/N)	Status/Comments

Site-Visit Report

The site-visit report gathers information about the program components and their level of implementation (Table 12.9).

Journal Entries

Journal entries were based on a template provided by the evaluation team. The items for the journal entries were

- number of minutes on exercise equipment per day

- number of minutes walking with peer per day

- number of calories consumed per day

- food intake per day—quantity and type

- use of problem-solving skills to control food intake and to exercise regularly

Attendance Sheet

The attendance sheet (Table 12.10) was used to gather information about participants in all the community-based events both on- and off-site. It is a record of the number of people who attended the events, and it provides a list of people who could be contacted for future evaluations. In addition the list could be used to provide a data base for promoting the initiative's activities and for distributing the community survey. It provides information about the reach of the program over time.

Record Review Sheet

The record review sheet records recommendations and actions related to the initiative components from board and committee meetings. It includes the date of the review, the title/name of the document, the date of the document, and a summary of the document.

TABLE 12.10.   **Sample Attendance Sheet**

Name of Session: _____
Date: _____
Location: _____

Name	Mailing Address	Telephone Number	E-mail Address	Comments
Janet Hairington	334 Wilsden Avenue	358–648–1285	harrj@yahoo.com	

Staff and Participant Interviews

Staff and participant interviews were conducted annually. The first occurred six months after the initiative started. The intent was to understand the programs that were being offered and to elicit recommendations for the annual report. Staff and program participants were interviewed for approximately sixty minutes. The following questions were asked:

- What role do you play in the organization?

- What programs does the Healthy Soon Project offer?

- Who is being served by the program?

- What experiences most represent your feelings about this initiative?

- What do you value most about the program?

- What are the programs processes and successes so far?

- What three things do you especially wish for the program?

- What recommendations do you have for reducing the rate of diabetes among members of this community?

For program participants an additional question was, "Think back to the last six months and being in this program. Tell a story about your experience."

The data from the interviews were analyzed to identify themes using theoretical and empirical constructs embedded in the interview guide used for data collection. The qualitative software package NVivo® was used to code the qualitative-data transcripts.

Survey

In order to determine whether the intervention had made a difference to the women participating compared with the women who were in the control group, a variety of data were collected. To assess the long-term outcome of the initiative—to increase the proportion of African American women who participate in the intervention who are at a healthy weight to 60 percent by 2012—the evaluators used laboratory tests, surveys, in-depth interviews, and journal reviews to assess knowledge, attitudes, and behavior with regard to diabetes and its prevention at baseline, after the first six weeks, and again one year later.

Among other items, the surveys assessed

- demographics (age, income, education level, family size, residence, zip code)
- knowledge of diabetes
- knowledge of risk factor for diabetes
- knowledge of the value of physical activity in preventing diabetes
- knowledge of the value of good nutrition in preventing diabetes
- attitudes towards getting diabetes
- perceptions of alcohol advertising in convenience stores
- levels of physical activity
- consumption of fruits and vegetables as part of a meal
- use of convenience stores
- use of farmers' markets

A fifty-item survey was developed from specifically made-up items and previously developed items. The compiled survey was reviewed by all the members of the evaluation team and then sent out to four independent reviewers for their expert opinion. It was reviewed by the Institutional Review Board and pilot-tested with a sample of thirty African American women.

The final survey was distributed as part of the project registration to serve as the baseline and again one year later for the intervention and the comparison groups. Women in both the intervention and the comparison groups were asked to complete the survey. All surveys were completed in an average of twenty minutes.

Three statements were included in the survey. The statements "Regular exercise helps to prevent diabetes," and "Good nutrition helps to prevent diabetes" were responded to on a five-point scale from "strongly disagree" to "strongly agree." The statement "It is okay for people to get diabetes" had a dichotomous yes/no response.

ANALYZE AND INTERPRET THE DATA

Site Visit

Quality Evaluation Inc. conducted a site visit to determine the status of the project components two weeks after the start of the initiative. The women in the intervention group had completed a baseline assessment; they were attending the prescribed number of sessions at the gym, which was fully equipped; and they had their initial meeting with the dietician. In addition, participants recruited a relative or friend to walk with them every evening. Each participant had completed the initial screening tests and was required to complete a journal. The baseline data and the screening tests were also completed for the comparison group. The records kept by the organization indicated that fifty African American women were enrolled in the study and another fifty were enrolled into the comparison group.

Work toward developing the alcohol-advertising legislation had started with a review of existing laws and the development of the legal and regulatory framework. An advocacy coalition had formed that brought together a group of ten advocates. Farmers had been contacted to develop the farmers' market. The site was being located, and permits were being obtained. A training was being planned and scheduled for the convenience store owners who had agreed to participate in the project, and monthly meetings were being held to facilitate the development of the convenience store initiative.

The site visit was conducted by two independent teams from Quality Evaluations Inc., using a protocol with predefined terms and categories for assessment. Each team consisted of an experienced evaluator and a member of the community. The results of each assessment were compared, comments were compiled, and discrepancies were resolved against standards that had been determined previously. For example, the standard for "fully implemented" had been previously defined by the team as being implemented exactly as defined by the protocol. Standards were defined in consultation with the CAPHO executive director because slight changes had been made since the original plans had been written. Table 12.11 is the site-visit report filled out by one of the evaluation teams.

Survey

There were fifty participants in the intervention group and fifty in the comparison group when they completed the survey at baseline. Their ages were comparable, with a mean age of 46.9 years, and the educational level of both groups was a mean of 8.6 years. A few had completed high school (10 percent), and none had gone to college. They worked in the service industry and many traveled to the nearby beaches to work. The intervention group lived in one of two zip code areas with the highest poverty level in the county, and the comparison group lived in the other. The average income of the intervention group was $6,900 per year, and the average income for the comparison group was $ 7,240. They were separated by the River Rokel, which is six miles wide. Most (75 percent) had children between the ages of six and eighteen years living at home.

TABLE 12.11. **Site-Visit Report at Two Weeks**

Name of Component	Fully Implemented (Y/N)	Participants Registered (Y/N)	Status/Comments
Physical activity in gym	Y	Y	Gym equipped, open daily for eight hours, staffed by two certified trainers, fifty participants in each group registered, baseline measures taken; journal entries
Nutrition	Y	Y	Dietician hired, available twenty hours per week, session length of one hour, fifty participants in each group registered, baseline measures taken; journal entries
Walking with peers	Y	Y	All intervention participants paired; journal entries
Legal and regulatory framework developed	N		Existing laws reviewed, coalition formed, meetings held quarterly with legislators, monthly newsletter
Farmers' markets	N		Farmers contacted, establishing schedule, site located
Convenience store initiative	N		Monthly meetings scheduled, minutes taken, trainer identified, training scheduled
CAPHO/farmers/ store owners partnership developed	N		Monthly meetings scheduled, minutes taken

Women in both the intervention group and the comparison group were given journals to complete at baseline. Two weeks into the project, journals were being completed as prescribed by the intervention group. The initial assessment was that the journals were being completed daily. Individual interviews with staff revealed that the intervention was being implemented as described in the protocols.

Only 15 percent of the intervention group and 20 percent of the comparison group was at a healthy weight, and all met the criteria for prediabetes with marginally high blood glucose levels. Only 15 percent exercised for approximately thirty minutes per week.

The mean scores for knowledge of the value of physical activity in preventing diabetes was 2.86 for the intervention group and 3.06 for the comparison group. For the question about knowledge of the value of nutrition in preventing diabetes, the mean score for the intervention group was 2.96, while the mean score for the comparison group was 3.02 (Table 12.12). Neither of the differences in scores was significant.

When participants were asked about their attitude toward diabetes, 36 percent of the intervention group said it was okay for people to get diabetes, while in the comparison group 34 percent said it was okay (Table 12.13). These data are comparable.

Interpretation

The data showed that the critical components of the initiative were fully implemented and less critical components were not yet implemented in the first month of the initiative. For instance, the six-week exercise/nutrition initiative was fully staffed, participants were recruited for both the intervention group and the control group, and appropriate measurements were being taken. The baseline data revealed no significant

TABLE 12.12.   **Intervention Group and Control Group at Baseline on Knowledge About Physical Activity and Nutrition**

Item	Intervention Group (mean)	Comparison Group (mean)	Significance
Physical activity	2.86	3.06	.619
Nutrition	2.96	3.02	.633

TABLE 12.13.   **Intervention Group and Control Group at Baseline on Attitude Toward Diabetes**

Response Category	Intervention Group (%)	Comparison Group (%)
Yes	18 (36)	17 (34)
No	32 (64)	33 (66)
Total	50 (100)	50 (100)

difference between the intervention and the comparison groups. However, approximately a third of individuals in both the intervention group (36 percent) and the comparison group (34 percent) reported not being concerned about getting diabetes, a finding that suggests considerable effort must be devoted to the educational component.

The farmers' market and the convenience store initiatives had not yet been implemented. Meetings had begun among the constituencies, and a coordinator had been named, ensuring that the remaining components were being developed.

The initial study conducted by Quality Evaluation Inc. was to determine whether the preliminary findings indicated that the intervention was likely to produce the anticipated outcomes. Although the study was conducted too early to provide a definitive answer with regard to the outcome, the critical components were in place and the protocols were being followed. The initial samples indicated that the target population group was registered to participate, and baseline laboratory readings suggested, based on evidence from existing research, that the anticipated outcome of a healthy weight could be attained. The team expected they would be able to demonstrate the value of the intervention to the community in lower rates of diabetes risk factors and indicators among those who participated compared to the comparison group, and to replicate the project to reach many more women in the succeeding years. They expected that in the years to come they would reduce the incidence of diabetes as well.

REPORT THE RESULTS

Quality Evaluation Inc. knew that the executive director and the staff would be interested in knowing how they were doing and wanted to provide feedback to the evaluation team. In consultation with the executive director and the staff, they decided that for this first report they would have forty-five minutes of the regular monthly staff meeting to present their findings. The reporting was evenly divided between the original members of the team and the stakeholders who had joined the team. It was an exciting time for them because it was their first evaluation. The team developed a short report and some table and charts; they gave an oral presentation from a set of PowerPoint slides and answered questions. After the presentation, they discussed the evaluation team's findings and next steps. The evaluation team completed the report with the feedback they received and sent the executive director a copy for her records.

During the meeting, three recommendations were added to the list the evaluation team already had. They were all adopted immediately. The most critical was to make sure sufficient educational materials were available for the women. Antoinette had recently found out about a set of materials about prediabetes, so they decided it would be a worthwhile purchase for the organization. Women in the intervention group were provided the additional materials. The other recommendations were ensuring that the farmers' market and convenience store components were fully implemented.

An analysis of the evaluation process showed that the team had been able to complete the tasks it had outlined; and they were satisfied they would be able to draw defensible conclusions about the Healthy Soon Project. They would make periodic checks to make sure the data were being collected and to provide any technical assistance that was needed. The team analyzed the data from the intervention and provided appropriate reports of the findings. Through a foundation grant to expand the program, Antoinette's team was able to provide evaluation services to the organization for five years.

GLOSSARY

Accuracy Standard of evaluation practice that requires that an evaluation be conducted by applying accurate and systematic processes.

Activities The specific initiative components that participants will take part in or be exposed to and that will result in products and changes to the participants.

Activity objective Specification of the activities necessary for carrying out the initiative.

Attrition threats to internal validity The loss of participants in an intervention that is different from the loss that occurs in the initially similar comparison group.

Behavioral objective Specification of the behavior that needs to be modified to achieve an outcome objective.

Community A group of people who live within a geographically confined area such as a block, a neighborhood, a town, or a village, or a group of people with similar interests.

Community assessment A description of the perceived and actual needs, assets, and resources of a given population that can be used in the development of a public health initiative.

Community-Based Participatory Research An approach and a philosophy for conducting research that both encourages power sharing and empowers community members.

Community health The health of people within a community.

Community organization A community-driven process for addressing health and social problems.

Consent forms Forms that contain information about a research study, the risks involved, the voluntary nature of the study, and the confidentiality of patient information. These forms specify the benefits of participating and provide contact information for an independent institutional representative whom the study participant can get in touch with if necessary.

Construct validity The extent to which a measure is theoretically sound.

Content validity The extent to which the items in an instrument are well defined.

Cost-benefit, or cost-effectiveness, analysis An assessment of the costs and benefits associated with an initiative and a determination of the value of expenditures.

Cross-cultural communication Approaches for understanding words and expressions and the use of language in communicating across cultures.

Cultural competence Knowledge, attitudes, and values that, when applied systematically, lead to the empowerment of others irrespective of their culture.

Culture The beliefs, traditions, and behavior of a group of people as observed in personal characteristics, geographical area, or common interests.

Data-coding and data-analysis software Software used to code and analyze text-based data in qualitative research with tools such as NVivo,® N6® from QSR, Ethnograph,® ATLASti,® and ANSWR.

Data-management tools Tables and charts that provide a template for outlining tasks and responsibilities and devising records for decision making.

Demographic Information about the fundamental characteristics of a given population.

Ecological model A model that describes the interpersonal, community, institutional, and public-policy influences on individual health behavior.

Ethical principles in program evaluation American Evaluation Association ethical values of systematic inquiry, competence, integrity/honesty, and responsibility for general and public welfare.

Ethnography Research that describes social change and allows increased understanding of different social cultures.

Evaluation standards Standards for utility, feasibility, propriety, and accuracy.

Executive summary A one- to two-page synopsis of an evaluation report.

Experimental design A rigorous research design that compares a randomly assigned control group to the intervention group in order to produce defensible conclusions that the intervention caused the changes that occurred.

External validity The extent to which an observed effect (outcome) can be generalized to other settings and to other populations.

Feasibility Standard of evaluation practice that requires that an evaluation process be practical.

Fidelity Implementation of an initiative as intended by a plan.

Formative evaluation An evaluation implemented at the very beginning of a project or to assess whether the fully implemented initiative is likely to have the intended effect.

Goal A stated desire to meet an expressed and unmet population need; provides direction for the initiative.

Health/program (or program/health) objective Specification of the overall direction of an initiative for addressing a public health problem.

Health Belief Model A theory based on individuals' perceptions of the problem and the benefits, barriers, and factors influencing the decision to adopt a behavior.

History threats to internal validity Events that take place outside the intervention but that affect the changes that are assessed.

Hypothesis A prediction of how an intervention would work under specific conditions.

Impact The benefit of an initiative in accomplishing a public health goal.

Impact evaluation Assessment of the effect at the population level of multiple initiatives.

Implementation Putting an initiative into effect according to a definite plan or specified procedure.

Indicator The quantitative or qualitative variable that allows changes that occur as a result of an intervention to be measured.

Informed consent A description of a program, its risks, and its benefits that allows an individual to make a decision about participating.

Initiative A program or policy intervention that addresses a health or social concern.

Inputs The human, financial, and material resources that are used for an initiative.

Institutional Review Board (IRB) A formally constituted committee designated to review, approve, and monitor biomedical and behavioral research that involves human subjects.

Instrumentation threats to internal validity Changes that occur in the measurement tools used to assess the effect of a program.

Internal validity The extent to which an achieved effect is due to a systematically planned intervention.

Interval-level data Data points where the distances between the points have real meaning. For example, the difference between eighty degrees and ninety degrees is the same ten degrees as the difference between sixty degrees and seventy degrees.

Literature review An integrated summary of existing reports of research and practice.

Logic model A brief summary of a program theory in simple or complicated illustrative and diagrammatic form.

Maturation threats to internal validity Changes in the study participants that are due to natural and physiological development that takes place over time.

Mobilizing for Action through Planning and Partnerships (MAPP) A process that consists of assessments of a local public health system, community themes and strengths, forces for change, and community health status.

Nominal-level data Data points that allow for a distinction in categories that are mutually exclusive, such as gender (male/female).

Objective A statement of how a goal will be achieved; it provides the initiative's precise direction and defines its planned purposes. Objectives are short, intermediate, or long term, and there are different types—health/program, behavioral, outcome, and activity objectives.

Observational, or nonexperimental, designs Evaluation designs that have neither a baseline nor a comparison or control group.

Ordinal-level data Data points that reflect a rank order within categories but have no meaning other than the indication of a rank order.

Outcome A change that occurs for the participants in a program or those who are exposed to a policy.

Outcome evaluation The determination of the effect of a program or policy on the beneficiaries of the initiative.

Outcome objective Specification for how the behavioral objective will be achieved; it is written at one or more of five areas of influence: individual, interpersonal, organizational, community, public policy.

Outputs The initial products of an initiative; they are generally a result of the intervention.

Participatory Model for Evaluation An approach to evaluation that adopts community-based participatory-research principles that embrace the stakeholders as co-learners.

Pilot testing Determination of whether an instrument or program works under real-life conditions and especially whether it works well in the population for which it is intended.

Population sampling Strategy to ensure appropriate representation of the population of interest in a sampling frame that is based on either probability or nonprobability sampling.

Preassessment A feasibility study of an initiative's readiness to be evaluated.

Primary data Information collected for the purposes of a particular study.

Process evaluation An assessment of the extent to which a program is being implemented as planned.

Program activities The specific initiative components that participants will participate in or be exposed to that will result in products and changes in the participants.

Program goal Specification of the overall direction of an initiative for addressing a public health problem.

Propriety Standard of evaluation practice that requires that an evaluation be ethical and conducted with regard for the rights of those involved and affected.

Protective factors Personal and environmental factors or determinants that protect against disease or disability.

Qualitative data Data collected with the use of narrative and observational approaches to understand individuals' knowledge, perceptions, attitudes, and behavior.

Quantitative data Numerical data collected to understand individuals' knowledge, understanding, perceptions, and behavior.

Quasi-experimental design A rigorous research design that compares a nonrandomly assigned comparison group to the intervention group in order to provide defensible conclusions that the intervention caused the changes that occurred.

Ratio-level data Data points that provides a true zero. Length, height, and age are good examples.

Regression threats to internal validity If study participants are selected on the basis of high or low baseline scores, the results of the testing will show they regress toward the population mean.

Risk factors Personal and environmental factors or determinants that increase the likelihood of an individual coming into contact with or being exposed to conditions that lead to disease or disability.

Saturation The point during qualitative data collection when the same information is being gathered from interviewees.

Secondary data Information collected for a previous purpose.

Selection threats to internal validity Differences in a study population between the intervention and the comparison group.

SMART Acronym for the characteristics of well developed program and policy initiative objectives—specific, measurable, attainable, realistic, and time-oriented.

Social Cognitive Theory A theory that hypothesizes that personal factors, environmental factors, and individual behavior operate in a dynamic, reciprocal way.

Social Support Theory A theory based on individuals' perception and experience of support from those around them.

SPSS® A type of quantitative-analysis software.

Stakeholders Individuals who have an interest in a program's development, implementation, or results.

Statistical-conclusion threats to internal validity Threats caused by the sample size being too small to show the effect and/or the measurement instruments being unstable and unlikely to measure true changes because of high standard-error estimates.

Testing threats to internal validity Changes that occur to the study participants when a test is given before the intervention that may affect the results positively or negatively when given again after the intervention in pre/post–test designs.

Theory of Planned Behavior A theory that hypothesizes the relationship between individuals' intentions, attitudes, and perceptions of social norms and their ability to perform a behavior.

Theory of Change A theory that hypothesizes clear and logical links among a program's mission, goal, objectives, and activities.

Threats to internal validity Characteristics that undermine the ability of a program to demonstrate a causal effect. These threats include attrition, history, instrumentation, maturation, regression, selection, statistical-conclusion validity, and testing.

Transtheoretical Model A model based on individuals' changing behavior through stages of readiness.

Triangulation Use of multiple data sources and data-collection approaches to increase cross-checking, substantiate findings, and increase validity.

Type I error Erroneously drawing the conclusion that an intervention had an impact on the intervention group and not the control or comparison group when, in fact, the intervention group and the control group did not differ.

Type II error Erroneously drawing the conclusion that the intervention had no impact when in fact it did and the results for the intervention group should have been different from the results for the control or comparison group.

Utility Standard of evaluation practice that requires that the information provided by an evaluation be useful to the stakeholders and those who will use the results.

REFERENCES

Abbatangelo-Gray, J., Cole, G. E., & Kennedy, M. G. (2007). Guidance for evaluating mass communication health initiatives: Summary of an expert panel discussion sponsored by the Centers for Disease Control and Prevention. *Evaluation & the Health Professions 30*, 229–253.

American Evaluation Association. (2008). Guiding principles for evaluators. *American Journal of Evaluation 29*(3), 233–234.

Andersen, R. M. (1995). Revisiting the behavioral model and access to medical care: Does it matter? *Journal of Health and Social Behavior 36*(1), 1–10.

Babbie, E. (1990). *Survey Research Methods.* Belmont, CA: Wadsworth.

Bandura, A. (1986). *Social Foundations of Thought and Action: A Social Cognitive Theory.* Englewood Cliffs, NJ: Prentice Hall.

Batancourt, J. R., Green, A. R., Carillo, J. E., & Ananeh-Firenpong, O. (2003). Defining cultural competence. A practical framework for addressing racial/ethnic disparities in health and health care. *Public Health Reports 118*, 293–302.

Belcher, H. J. (1994). *Group Participation.* 2nd ed. Thousand Oaks, CA: Sage.

Bender, D. E., & Harbour, C. (2001). Tell me what you mean by "si": Perceptions of quality of prenatal care among immigrant Latina women. *Qualitative Health Research 1*(6), 780–794.

Carmines, E., & Zeller, R. A. (1979). *Reliability and Validity Assessment,* vol. 07-017. Thousand Oaks, CA: Sage.

Centers for Disease Control and Prevention. (1999). *Framework for Program Evaluation in Public Health.* Atlanta: Centers for Disease Control and Prevention.

Centers for Disease Control and Prevention. (rev.: November 30, 2007). *Tiers of Evidence: A framework for classifying HIV behavioral interventions.* Retrieved June 18, 2009, from www.cdc.gov/hiv/topics/research/prs/print/tiers-of-evidence.htm

Cohen, J. (1960). A coefficient of agreement for nominal scales. *Educational and Psychological Measurement 20*, 37–46.

Commission on Social Determinants of Health. (2008). *Closing the Gap in a Generation: Health Equity Through Action on the Social Determinants of Health. Final Report of the Commission on Social Determinants of Health.* Geneva: World Health Organization.

Cook, T. D., & Campbell, D. T. (1979). *Quasi-experimentation: Design and Analysis Issues for Field Settings.* Chicago: Rand McNally.

Cooper, C., P., Jorgensen, C. M., & Meritt, T. L. (2003). Report from the CDC. Telephone focus groups: An emerging method in public health research. *Journal of Women's Health 12*(10), 945–951.

Creswell, J. W. (2007). *Qualitative Inquiry and Research Design. Choosing Among Five Approaches.* 2nd ed. Thousand Oaks, CA: Sage.

Daponte, B. O. (2008). *Evaluation Essentials. Methods for Conducting Sound Research.* San Francisco: Jossey-Bass.

David, A. J. (2005). Enhancing quality of practice through Theory of Change-Based Evaluation: Science or practice? *American Journal of Community Psychology 35*(3–4), 159–168.

Delbecq, A. L., Van de Ven, A. H., & Gustafson, D. H. (1975). *Group Techniques for Program Planning.* Glenview, IL: Scott, Foresman.

Dillman, D. A. (2000). *Mail and Internet Survey: The Tailored Design Method.* New York: Wiley.

Fazlay, F. S., Lofton, S. P., Doddato, T. M., & Mangum, C. (2003). Utilizing Geographic Information Systems in community assessment and nursing research. *Journal of Community Health Nursing 20*(3), 179–191.

Fern, E. (2001). *Advanced Focus Group Research.* Thousand Oaks, CA: Sage.

Fetterman, D. M., Kaftarian, S. J., & Wandersman, A. (1996). *Empowerment Evaluation: Knowledge and Tools for Self-Assessment and Accountability.* Thousand Oaks, CA: Sage.

Feveile, H., Olsen, O., & Hugh, A. (2007). A randomized trial of mailed questionnaires versus telephone interviews. Response patterns in a survey. *BMC Medical Research Methodology 7*(27), 1–7.

Finifter, D. H., Jensen, C. J., Wilson, C. E., & Koenig, B. L. (2005). A comprehensive, multitiered, targeted community needs assessment model. *Family & Community Health 28,* 293–306.

Fishbain, M., & Ajzen, I. (1975). *Belief, Attitude, Intention and Behavior: An Introduction to Theory and Research.* Reading, MA: Addison-Wesley.

Fitzpatrick, J. L., Sanders, J. R., & Worthen, B. R. (2004). *Program Evaluation. Alternative Approaches and Practical Guidelines.* 3rd ed. Boston: Pearson.

Frechtling, J. A. (2007). *Logic Modeling Methods in Program Evaluation.* San Francisco: Jossey-Bass.

Ghere, G., King, J. A., Stevahn, L., & Minnema, J. (2006). A professional development unit for reflecting on program evaluator competencies. *American Journal of Evaluation, 27,* 108–123.

Giacomini, M. K., & Cook, D. J. (2000). Users' guide to the medical literature: XXIII. Qualitative research in health care. Are the results of the study valid? *Journal of the American Medical Association 284*(3), 357–362.

Glanz, K., & National Cancer Institute (U.S.). (2005). *Theory at a Glance: A Guide for Health Promotion Practice.* 2nd ed. Bethesda, MD: National Cancer Institute, U.S. Department of Health and Human Services.

Glanz, K., Rimer, B. K., & Viswanath, K. (2008). The scope of health behavior and health education. In *Health Behavior and Health Education: Theory, Research and Practice,* 4th ed., ed. K. Glanz, B. K. Rimer, & K. Viswanath, 3–22. San Francisco: Jossey-Bass.

Hancock, T., & Minkler, M. (2007). Community health assessment or healthy community assessment. Whose community? Whose health? Whose assessment? In *Community Organizing and Community Building for Health,* 3rd ed., ed. M. Minkler, 138–157. New Brunswick, NJ: Rutgers University Press.

Harris, M., & López-Defede, A. (2004). *Understanding the Social and Cultural Determinants of Tuberculosis: A South Carolina Study.* Columbia, SC: Institute for Families in Society.

Hochbaum, G. M. (1958). *Participation in Medical Screening Programs: A Psychological Study.* Washington, DC: U.S. Department of Health, Education and Medicine.

House, J. S. (1981). *Work, Stress and Social Support.* Reading, MA: Addison-Wesley.

Institute of Medicine. (2001). *The Future of Public Health.* Washington, DC: Institute of Medicine.

Israel, B. A., Eng, E., Schulz, A. J., & Parker, E. A., eds. (2005). *Methods in Community-Based Participatory Research for Health.* San Francisco: Jossey-Bass.

Jekel, J. F., Elmore, J. G., & Katz, D. L. (1996). *Epidemiology, Biostatistics and Preventive Medicine.* Philadelphia: Saunders.

Johnson, E. C., Kirkhart, K. E., Madison, A. M., Noley, G. B., & Solano-Flores, G. (2008). The impact of narrow views of scientific rigor on evaluation practices for underrepresented groups. In *Fundamental Issues in Evaluation,* ed. N. L. Smith & P. R. Brandon, 261. New York: Guilford Press.

Joint Committee on Standards for Educational Evaluation, Sanders, J. R., & American Association of School Administrators. (1994). *The Program Evaluation Standards: How to Assess Evaluations of Educational Programs.* 2nd ed. Thousand Oaks, CA: Sage.

Keiffer, E. C., Salabarria-Pena, Y., Odoms-Young, A. M., Willis, S. K., Baber, K. E., & Gusman, J. R. (2005). The application of focus group methodologies to Community Based Participatory Research. In *Methods in Community-Based Participatory Research for Health,* ed. B. A. Israel, E. Eng, A. J. Schulz, & E. A. Parker, 146–166. San Francisco: Jossey-Bass.

King, J. A., Stevahn, L., Ghere, G., & Minnema, J. (2001). Toward a taxonomy of essential evaluator competencies. *American Journal of Evaluation 22*(2), 229–248.

Kirkhart, K. E. (2005). Through a cultural lens: Reflections on validity and theory in evaluation. In *The Role of Culture and Cultural Context: A Mandate for Inclusion, the Discovery of Truth, and Understanding in Evaluative Theory and Practice*, ed. S. Hood, R. Hopson, & H. Frierson, 21–39. Greenwich, CT: IAP- Information Age Publishing.

Kretzmann, J. P., & McKnight, J. L. (1993). *Building Communities from the Inside Out: A Path Towards Finding and Mobilizing a Community's Assets*. Evanston, IL: Center for Urban Affairs and Policy Research.

Krueger, R. A., & Casey, M. A. (2000). *Focus Groups*. 3rd ed. Thousand Oaks, CA: Sage.

Marmot, M. (2004). *The Status Syndrome*. New York: Henry Holt.

Mason, J. (2002). *Qualitative Researching*. 2nd ed. Thousand Oaks, CA: Sage.

Maxwell, J. A. (2005). *Qualitative Research Design. An Interactive Approach*. 2nd ed. Thousand Oaks, CA: Sage.

McLennan, E., Strotman, R., McGregor, J., & Dolan, D. (2004). AnSWR users guide. Retrieved Oct. 19. 2008, from http://www.cdc.gov/hiv/topics/surveillance/resources/software/answr/index.htm

Milstein, B., Wetterhall, S., & Group, C.E.W. (2000). A framework featuring steps and standards for program evaluation. *Health Promotion Practice 1*(3), 221–228.

Minkler, M., ed. (2007). *Community Organizing and Community Building for Health*. 3rd ed. New Brunswick, NJ: Rutgers University Press.

Minkler, M., Wallerstein, N., & Wilson, N. (2008). Improving health through community organization and community building. In *Health Behavior and Health Education: Theory, Research and Practice*, 4th ed., ed. K. Glanz, B. K. Rimer, & K. Viswanath, 287–312. San Francisco: Jossey-Bass.

National Association of County and City Health Officials (n.d.). Mobilizing for Action Through Planning and Partnerships. Retrieved Sept. 20, 2009, from http://www.naccho.org/topics/infrastructure/MAPP/index.cfm

Nelson-Barber, S., LeFrance, J., Trumbull, E., & Aburto, S. (2005). Promoting culturally reliable and valid evaluation practice. In *The Role of Culture and Cultural Context: A Mandate for Inclusion, the Discovery of Truth and Understanding in Evaluative Theory and Practice*, ed. S. Hood, R. Hopson, & H. Frierson, 61–85. Greenwich, CT: IAP-Information Age Publishing.

O'Fallon, L., & Dearry, A. (2002). Community-based participatory research as a tool to advance environmental health sciences. *Environmental Health Perspectives 110* (supplement 2), 155–159.

Panet-Raymond, J. (1992). Partnership myth or reality? *Community Development Journal 27*(2), 156–165.

Patton, M. Q. (2008). *Utilization-Focused Evaluation*. 4th ed. Thousand Oaks, CA: Sage.

Perez, M. A., & Luquis, R. R. (2008). *Cultural Competence in Health Education and Health Promotion*. San Francisco: Jossey-Bass.

Preskill, H., & Catsambas, T. T. (2006). *Reframing Evaluation Through Appreciative Inquiry*. Thousand Oaks, CA: Sage.

Procashasca, J. O., & DiClemente, C. C. (1983). Stages and processes of self change of smoking: Towards an integrative model of change. *Journal of Counselling and Clinical Psychology 51*, 390–395.

Public Health Leadership Society. (2002). *Principles of the Ethical Practice of Public Health*. New Orleans: Public Health Leadership Society.

Rappaport, J. (1984). Studies in empowerment: Introduction to the issue. *Prevention in Human Services 3*(2–3), 1–7.

Rossi, P. H., Lipsey, M. W., & Freeman, H. E. (2004). *Evaluation. A Systematic Approach*. Thousand Oaks, CA: Sage.

Russell, L. B., Siegal, J. E., Daniels, N., Gold, M. R., Luce, B. R., & Mandelblatt, J. S. (1997). Cost-effectiveness analysis as a guide to resource allocation in health: Roles and limitation. In *Cost-Effectiveness in Health and Medicine*, ed. M. R. Gold, J. E. Siegel, L. B. Russell, M. C. Weinstein, 3–24. New York: Oxford University Press.

Sallis, J. F., Owen, N., & Fisher, E. B. (2008). Ecological models of health behavior. In *Health Behavior and Health Education: Theory, Research and Practice*, ed. K. Glanz, B. K. Rimer, & K. Viswanath, 465–482. San Francisco: Jossey-Bass.

Savage, C. L., Xu, Y., Lee, R., Rose, B. L., Kappesser, M., & Anthony, J. S. (2006). A case study in the use of Community Based Participatory Research in public health nursing. *Public Health Nursing 23*(5), 472–478.

Schulz, A. J., Zenk, S. N., Kannan, S., Israel, B. A., Koch, M. A., & Stokes, C. A. (2005). CBPR approach to survey design and implementation. In *Methods in Community-Based Participatory Research for Health,* ed. B. A. Israel, E. Eng, A. J. Schulz, & E. A. Parker, 107–127. San Francisco: Jossey-Bass.

Sector, R. E. (1995). *Cultural Diversity in Health and Illness.* 4th ed. Stamford, CT: Appleton & Lang.

Sharpe, P. A., Greany, M. L., Lee, P. R., & Royce, S. W. (2005). Assets-oriented community assessment. *Public Health Reports 115,* 205–211.

Shi, L. (2008). *Health Services Research Methods.* 2nd ed. Clifton Park, NY: Thomson/Delmar Learning.

Stufflebeam, D. L., & Shinkfield, A. J. (2007). *Evaluation Theory, Models, and Applications.* San Francisco: Jossey-Bass.

Substance Abuse and Mental Health Administration. (2008). National Registry of Evidence-Based Programs and Practices. Retrieved Sept. 20, 2009, from http://www.nrepp.samhsa.gov/find.asp

Tervalon, M., & Murray-Garcia, J. (1998). Cultural humility vs. cultural competence. A critical distinction in defining physician training outcomes in medical education. *Journal of Health Care for the Poor and Underserved 9*(2), 117–125.

Travers, R., Wilson, M. G., Flicker, S., Guta, A., Bereket, T., McKay, C., et al. (2008). The greater involvement of people living with AIDS principle: Theory versus practice in Ontario's HIV/AIDS community-based research sector. *AIDS Care 20*(6), 615–624.

Ulin, P. R., Robinson, E. T., & Tolley, E. E. (2005). *Qualitative Methods in Public Health: A Field Guide for Applied Research.* San Francisco: Jossey-Bass.

United Nations. (2008). *The Millennium Development Goals Report 2008.* New York: United Nations.

United Nations Population Fund. (n.d.). Guide to working from within; 24 tips for culturally sensitive programming. Retrieved Apr. 18, 2009, from http://www.unfpa.org/culture/24/cover.htm

U.S. Department of Health and Human Services. (Nov. 2000). *Healthy People 2010.* 2nd ed. 2 vols. Washington, DC: U.S. Government Printing Office.

Veach, R. M. (1997). *Medical Ethics.* 2nd ed. Studbury, MA: Jones & Bartlett.

Wallerstein, N., & Burnstein, E. (1998). Empowerment education: Freire's ideas adapted to health education. *Health Education Quarterly 15*(4), 379–394.

Wang, C., Burris, M. A., & Ping, X. Y. (1996). Chinese village women as visual anthropologists: A participatory approach to reaching policymakers. *Social Science & Medicine 42*(10), 1391–1400.

Windsor, R., Clark, N., Boyd, N. R., & Goodman, R. M. (2004). *Evaluation of Health Promotion, Health Education and Disease Prevention Programs.* 3rd ed. Boston: McGraw-Hill.

Zenk, S. N., Schulz, A. J., House, J. S., Benjamin, A., & Kannan, S. (2005). Application of CBPR in the design of an observational tool: The neighborhood observational checklist. In *Methods in Community-Based Participatory Research for Health,* ed. B. A. Israel, E. Eng, A. J. Schulz, & E. A. Parker, 167–187. San Francisco: Jossey-Bass.

INDEX

Page references followed by *fig* indicate an illustrated figure; followed by *t* indicate a table.

Printed in the United States of America
ED-02-04-13